Richard C. Sparks, C.S.P.

To Treat
or
Not To Treat

Bioethics and the Handicapped Newborn

PAULIST PRESS
New York/Mahwah

Index prepared by Michael Kerrigan, C.S.P.

Copyright © 1988 by
The Missionary Society
of St. Paul the Apostle
in the State of New York

Library of Congress Cataloging-in-Publication Data

Sparks, Richard C., 1950–
　　To treat or not to treat.

　　Includes bibliographies and index.
　　1. Neonatal intensive care—Moral and ethical aspects. 2. Infants (Newborn)—Diseases—Treatment—Moral and ethical aspects. 3. Neonatal intensive care—Decision-making. 4. Euthanasia—Moral and ethical aspects.
5. Medical ethics. I. Title.
RJ253.5.S62　　1988　　　174′.24　　　　88-9822
ISBN 0-8091-2993-0 (pbk.)

Published by Paulist Press
997 Macarthur Boulevard
Mahwah, New Jersey 07430

Printed and bound in the
United States of America

Table of Contents

Contents

INTRODUCTION

Between 1970 and 1980 the mortality rate among newborn infants in the United States was almost halved. Tiny infants, weighing 1,000 grams (2.2 pounds) or less, now have a reasonable chance of survival as compared with barely a ten percent possibility just two decades ago. The establishment in the 1960s of neonatology as a pediatric subspecialty and the creation of approximately six hundred Neonatal Intensive Care Units nationwide have contributed greatly to this lessening of infant mortality. Despite this technological progress, or in some cases partly because of it, still four percent of the infants born in this country annually are diagnosed as suffering from one or more readily detectable congenital abnormality.[1] In fact, recent statistics indicate that the number of babies born with some physical or mental defect has doubled over the past twenty-five years. The causes for this increase in handicaps among newborns are varied and far from clear. Theories include increased cigarette smoking among women, increased exposure to workplace toxins, and improved medical techniques that permit more children with disabilities to survive and, eventually, to pass the trait along in the gene pool to the next generation.[2]

For the parents of the 3–4 million so-called "normal" or healthy infants born in the U.S. each year, neonatology has been a blessing, in some cases a life-saver. For many of the infants rushed to an N.I.C.U., particularly those whose main problem is prematurity and/or low birth weight, initial respiratory problems, infections, jaundice, or feeding difficulties are only temporary. These medical problems are often completely "cured" through the use of ventilators, isolettes (no longer called incubators), gavage or I.V. feeding, and drug therapies. Time and patient care allow for most "premies" to develop extrauterine the organ systems left unrefined due to early birth.[3]

This somewhat "rosy" impression, however, is not intended

1

to gloss over the reality that for the vast majority of the nearly 150,000 infants annually born in this country with genetic, chromosomal, or environmentally-related anomalies, life will not be "normal."[4] Marshaling all the resources of modern medical technology in their behalf may in the end prove futile or may, as in the case of some respiratory and drug therapies, compound the handicap or even create new ones. The smaller the premature infant one salvages through resuscitation and ventilator therapy the greater the odds are that s/he will be destined for a lifetime of combat against one or more major medical handicaps. Similarly, prenatal and neonatal asphyxia and apnea as well as high grade (i.e. severe) intraventricular hemorrhages can, even if counteracted, permanently impair or even destroy brain, kidney, and intestinal functions. The variety, complexity, and interrelationship of congenital abnormalities and potential complications is beyond the scope of this present study. The table of contents of one standard text lists no fewer than 222 distinct deformities, acknowledging that roughly half of all handicapped newborns suffer from multiple other, as-yet-unnamed anomalies.[5]

In late 1963, at the Johns Hopkins Medical Center in Baltimore, an infant boy was born who lived for only fifteen days. The circumstances surrounding his brief life and the fact that he was the subject of a widely circulated 1972 film **Who Shall Survive?** have made the "Johns Hopkins Baby" one of a handful of well-known, ethically troubling cases regarding decisions not to treat handicapped or so-called "defective" newborns.[6] By some configuration or fluke of genetics this boy was that one in every 660 infants born with an extra chromosome at the twenty-first pairing—Trisomy 21, also known as Down's Syndrome. Physically, this congenital abnormality is marked by a relatively flat face, short neck, small head, slanted eyes (hence, the misnomer "Mongoloid"), stubby fingers, a simean-creased palm, and weak musculature. Mentally, such children are retarded, some severely, others only mildly so. One-third to one-half of all Trisomy

21 newborns suffer from one or more complicating problems, such as congenital heart defects, a higher susceptibility to infections, or a blockage somewhere along the digestive system. Such was the case with the Johns Hopkins Baby, who had a bowel obstruction (duodenal atresia), which prevented the normal flow and digestion of food. Easily correctable by relatively routine surgery, the problem would, as a matter of course, be corrected in all "normal" newborns.

However, in the Hopkins case two decisions were made by the parents with the support and acquiescence of the medical team. First, permission was withheld for the surgery, presumably based on some determination about the undesirability of life with Trisomy 21. Second, since the child could not digest food in his present condition, the order was given not to attempt feeding by natural, gavage, or intravenous means, thus insuring death by starvation or related pneumonia. Kept warm and dry, but untreated and unfed, the baby died over a two week period from complications due to non-nutrition.

In 1982 an almost identical case in Bloomington, Indiana, resurfaced the ethical issues involved when treatment is withheld on a life-threatening but correctable condition based on the presence of another non-lethal but arguably burdensome handicap.[7] Fearful of the potential abuse such decisions have on the rights of mentally retarded citizens, the Department of Health and Human Services issued a set of guidelines, immediately dubbed the "Reagan Ruling" or the "Baby Doe Rule," prohibiting as discriminatory the withholding of treatment solely on the basis of mental deficiency. Court rulings, two subsequent revisions, and a 1984 amendment to the Child Abuse Prevention and Protection Act (of 1974) have not altered the basic thrust of these regulations, though the most recent versions are better nuanced and more carefully phrased.[8]

While in both the Hopkins and Bloomington cases the majority of commentators believe a disservice was done to the

3

handicapped infants involved by a premature or even prejudicial decision to withhold treatment, the story of Lance Steinhaus raises the potential countervailing injustice of forced overtreatment. On March 20, 1986, Lance Tyler Steinhaus was born. On April 23 and 24, barely five weeks later, the infant "suffered a fractured skull, severe brain damage, broken ribs and other injuries" at the hands of his abusive father. Although the baby was not "brain dead," because his brain stem continued to support spontaneous heart and lung functions, Lance was "unable to see or hear or have any conscious thoughts."[9]

If medical personnel would continue to administer antibiotics, intubate as needed, and resuscitate him following seizures, Lance could be "kept alive" indefinitely. If this child-abuse victim were kept alive, his father, Timothy Steinhaus, could be charged in a court of law only with two counts of first-degree assault. If, however, antibiotics were discontinued or a "no code" order were established forbidding future resuscitation, the baby would soon die and, quite possibly, his father would be charged with third-degree murder. Lance's future was entrusted to District Court Judge George Harrelson of Marshall, Minnesota, while his father's fate was turned over to a neighboring judge.

According to testimony given by Lance's physician, Dr. David Steinhorn, the baby appeared to be in a "permanent vegetative state," a coma-like condition from which a patient rarely emerges (only two recorded cases of partial recovery). Minnesota Citizens Concerned for Life and the United Handicapped Association alerted Lance's father and his attorney to the Baby Doe Rule and 1984 law, which, if strictly interpreted, would seem not to permit the cessation of further treatment.

All the parties directly involved acknowledged that Lance was "virtually brain dead." As Dr. Steinhorn testified, the infant's E.E.G. indicated that he was "as close as possible to being brain dead without being brain dead." Judge Harrelson was caught on the horns of a legal dilemma. The present law, admittedly written as a compromise in a highly charged political atmosphere, permits withholding treatment if the infant is either "brain dead" or "chronically and irreversibly comatose." Is being in a permanent vegetative state synonymous with being irreversibly comatose? If so, the mother's desire to cease all further therapy, allowing the infant to die, would seem to be legal as well as moral. However, if P.V.S. is not equivalent to irreversible coma, then legally Lance must continue to receive treatment, however futile, burdensome, and potentially inhumane.

Initially the judge ruled that treatment must be continued. After subsequent medical testimony by a pediatric neurologist, clarifying the extent of Lance's mental damage and future prognosis, the judge reversed his order, allowing a "do not resuscitate" (DNR) order to be imposed in Lance's best interest. Finally, after ten months of life, nine of those lived totally void of consciousness, Lance Steinhaus died, or, one might say, "finished dying." In a sincere effort to respect the life of this tragically abused newborn, and to forestall premature or possibly prejudicial judgments akin to those made against some moderately retarded infants, Lance had been forced to undergo five futile, arguably assaultive therapies—one major resuscitation and four intubations—prior to his being allowed to die naturally.

"To treat or not to treat?" is THE ethical question facing many parents in a variety of neonatal situations. Often the debate is reduced somewhat unfairly to two caricatured positions, "sanctity of life" versus "quality of life." These two positions need not and ought not be seen as mutually exclusive. Spanning the last two decades, from the Hopkins Case (1963) through the Bloomington Baby Doe Case (1982) to the recent case of Lance Steinhaus (1986), controversial court litigations have arisen when decisions are made to withhold consent for therapy based not strictly on the benefit or burden of the proposed treatment, but on a projected quality of life to be enjoyed or endured by the newborn patient.

It is generally assumed that bodily life is a good, a valuable state of existence to be preserved and prolonged. Thus, society surrounds the lives of its members with moral and legal safeguards and also provides some degree of medical assistance to promote this "respect life" premise. However, for the past four centuries medical ethicists have tended to balance off this abiding concern for life with some qualifications, some exceptional instances when the mere prolongation of basic biological "life" (respiration and circulation) may be counterproductive to the well-being or "life" of the patient as a whole, body-spirit person. What are these "exceptional instances"? When, if ever, can one say that nontreatment is the best option?

In recent decades the discovery and relatively routine use of sophisticated, non-curative procedures and equipment, which serve to prolong respiration and circulation artificially, led to precedent-setting ethical questions concerning the case-by-case benefit or not of their interminable use. The cases of infants are all the more troubling since they are at the beginning edge of life, with so much to lose if an erroneous decision, either to forge ahead or to stop, is made in their behalf. In short, as our technological skills develop to the point where almost every infant can be "saved" or maintained, in terms of basic bodily functions, is it ever morally permissible to decide that what CAN be done NEED NOT be done, perhaps even OUGHT NOT be done?

This present volume is offered as a thorough survey of the ethical literature regarding the treatment or nontreatment of handicapped newborns. It is important to note as we begin that a linguistic metamorphosis is underway in the field. Prior to the mid-1970s the literature tended to freely use the adjective "defective" to describe all newborns with genetic, chromosomal, or environmentally-rooted abnormalities. Since that time various scholars and organizations concerned with the plight of such individuals have taken umbrage at the apparently pejorative implications of the word "defective," and have substituted most often the phrase "handicapped newborn." Sensitive to the implications of the choice of language, I will use the label handicapped newborns or infants, with "defective" always placed in quotation marks if and when used.[10]

Ethical discussions regarding the withdrawal or withholding of medical treatment from non-competent patients must face four distinct questions:

1. In the absence of a freely-choosing, competent patient as moral agent, WHO DECIDES for the non-competent patient (the senile elderly, the permanently unconscious, the severely brain-damaged, or the handicapped infant)?

2. ON WHAT BASIS is the decision to forego or cease treatment made?

3. If one chooses to cease all therapeutic efforts, WHAT IS THE NEXT STEP? This involves two subquestions: What in the way of humane or nursing care does "nontreatment" entail? Secondly, if one decides that death arriving sooner rather than later is best, may one choose active or direct euthanasia to achieve that end faster, more cheaply, and more efficiently?

4. Taking into account these ethical dimensions, WHAT IS OR OUGHT TO BE the legal ramifications in terms of PUBLIC POLICY?

This volume will deal almost exclusively with the second of these four questions.

While the first question "Who decides?" has spawned a respectable amount of literature, this researcher subscribes to the thesis that no lone person has full freedom with reference to the rights and best interest of non-competent others. In the case of children, parents or legal guardians are and ought to be the primary arbiters of their charges' care and best interests. However, the attending physician and health care team are not passive recipients of familial orders. Bringing to bear their medical expertise, prior experience, and "bedside manner," health care professionals assist parents in deciding whether treatment is warranted or not. Likewise, the institution, through its administrative structures or infant care review committee, and the society, through its judiciary system, act as checks and balances, avenues of recourse if discrimination or abuse against the voiceless patient is suspected. In the case of handicapped newborns, who decides? This volume is written with the presumption that it is the parents or guardian, in cooperation with the health care professionals, who are the primary deciders, under the benevolently watchful gaze of institutional ethics committees and the society at large.[11]

It seems to me that the second question—"On what basis is the decision to forego or cease treatment made?"—is distinct from, though related to, the subsequent question of euthanasia or infanticide. While decisions to withhold or withdraw treatment (Q #2) are sometimes labeled "passive" or "indirect" euthanasia (Q #3), refusing to prolong life or ceasing to prolong an irreversible dying process (i.e., nontreatment) frequently constitutes a different species of act from a decision to directly kill or to terminate life by indirect means. Presuming that the two are synonymous leads some scholars surveyed here to advocate active infanticide in many of those cases where nontreatment seems viable. This book will deal almost exclusively with the raison d'être of nontreatment decisions, leaving questions about the morality or advisability of active infanticide or direct euthanasia for a subsequent study.[12] Only to the extent that a given nontreatment standard lends itself to the "wedge" or "slippery slope" argument for euthanasia will the possible ramifications of condoning active infanticide be considered.

Likewise, the decision as to what sort of humane care one owes a patient selected out for nontreatment is also an important topic. Numerous recent articles on the optional versus mandatory nature of I.V. or gavage feeding could be the basis for such a study. That too will be alluded to where appropriate, but consciously placed beyond the scope of our focus on question number two, the criteria for nontreatment decisions.[13]

Finally, the fourth question, that of public policy, will be skirted, but not ignored. While law is not and ought not be seen as synonymous with what is ethically right or wrong in a given situation, obviously there is a close connection. First, one must establish the ethical limits, both in terms of procedure and criteria, which a society espouses and will condone. Only then, can the community, through its legislatures and courts, decide public policy. Should the law be stricter than what might be ethical in a given situation? This would forestall potential abuse by those wishing to stretch the exception clauses at the fringes of the legal limits. Or should the law be looser, allowing for situational exceptions and more autonomomous decisions, with which the mainstream might disagree, but tolerate in the name of reasonable pluralism?[14]

In the case of nontreatment decisions related to handicapped newborns, the recent (1982–1986) flurry of activity, both by the Department of Health and Human Services and by the Congress, attests that public policy in this area is a pressing concern. While this volume will not take up the issue of law specifically, it is hoped that the spectrum of moral positions presented and critiqued here will assist those whose expertise and interest is law.[15]

This volume will focus on the ethical question: **On what basis is it moral to forego or cease further treatment for a handicapped newborn?** A careful survey and analysis of the literature yields a spectrum of opinion concerning treatment questions regarding handicapped newborns. This spectrum can be subdivided more or less neatly into a fourfold typology, which will serve as the structural outline for this volume. It is designed to offer the reader a way of comprehending the ethical continuum. In many respects the ethical issues are identical to those involved in decisions to cease or forego treatment for non-competent adults like Karen Ann Quinlan, Joseph Saikewicz, or Brother Fox. However, the personal tragedy involved seems all the more poignant when the patient is newborn, at the starting edge of life, rather than at the end of a long or reasonably long life span. More importantly, adult non-competents, at some prior point in life, may have competently expressed wishes concerning such tragic life and death borderline situations. Their wishes rightly weigh heavily in final decisions now made for them by proxies. Handicapped infants, on the other hand, have never been competent, necessitating a wholly imputed or substituted judgment, based on the value system and intentionality of someone else, whether parents, physician, or society.

In each case it is a question of relating "benefit" to "burden," seeking some calculus of "net best interest." When is a given treatment, whether therapeutic or merely life-sustaining, considered a benefit? When, if ever, does such treatment itself become more of a deficit, an inordinate burden? Benefit and/or burden to whom? The patient alone? The patient's family? Society at large? Or some amalgam of all three? Is it ever a matter of one's life condition or "quality of life" being inordinately burdensome rather than the means causing such an imbalance? What about conflicts between the patient's medical or individual best interests and those of one's family or society?

These questions are fundamental and, in some sense, prior to particular case applications. So while various case scenarios dealing with anencephaly, spina bifida cystica, Trisomy 13, 18, and 21, duodenal atresia or esophageal fistula, Tay Sachs disease, and Lesch-Nyhan syndrome will appear in each chapter to illustrate the operation of that particular "type" or approach, the more fundamental issue to be explored will be the basis on which the decision is made. In no sense is this meant to be an exhaustive presentation of case applications. As noted earlier, the number of potential anomalies, combinations thereof, and situational complications defy all but the more generic comments, allowing for some situational prudence in applying one's ethical "type" or prioritized values to a given case.

At the far ends of the spectrum are two largely hypothetical positions for determining nontreatment, which will be noted here for theoretical completeness, but which will thereafter be presumed inadequate. At the far right or conservative end of the spectrum would be **absolute vitalism.** Accordingly, the physician is always obliged to treat and to sustain life "until the issue is taken out of his [her] hands."[16] Arguably, once placed on a respirator or ventilator one is destined to stay there either until one contracts some fatal non-respiratory condition or else the equipment "miraculously" shuts down of its own accord. Several scholars note that "the last serious advocate of this unconditional provitalist doctrine was David Karnofsky, the great tumor research scientist of the Sloan-Kettering Institute in New York."[17] More recently, well intentioned but unnuanced "Right to Life" activists and their impassioned apologists have bordered on advocating a vitalistic mandate never to cease treatment.[18] However, it is generally agreed by most ethicists and society at large that with the advent of mechanical life-sustaining equipment (respirators, heart pumps, pacemakers) there may rightly come times, however rare or frequent, when ceasing treatment or "pulling the plug" is a means of respecting human life, not harming it.

At the far left or liberal end of the spectrum would be an unbridled libertarian approach to nontreatment decisions. While some may advocate such **absolute autonomy,** allowing competent patients to accept or forego treatment at will, it is generally accepted by ethicists and by society that at least some, seemingly irrational or suicidal choices are beyond the pale, grounds for declaring the patient mentally "non-competent" to make such choices. In the case of non-competent patients, society generally condones some variations of a "reasonable person" standard, allowing the guardian to judge freely the best interest of the patient, provided s/he does not go wholly beyond the limits of what would generally or reasonably be deemed beneficial. To condone unrestrained autonomy is to simultaneously undercut the ethical enterprise itself. Absolute autonomy is a formal or procedural standard with no objective criteria. There are no longer right or wrong choices. Any decision, however relative or capricious, would seem permissible as long as the autonomous patient or guardian so chooses. Ethics would lose its prescriptive or ought-discerning role. If morality is reduced to a synonym for intentionality alone and if good will or even free whim is the measure of good acts, then subjectivism reigns and ethics becomes a lost art, a process without an anchor.

Between these two somewhat hypothetical poles, there is a moral spectrum that divides more or less neatly into four ethical standards or **types** with reference to the nontreatment of handicapped infants. By extension this typology seems applicable to all nontreatment decisions, but the focus of this present study will remain exclusively on the cases of handicapped newborns. The four types are:

   (1) A Medical Indications Policy (also called "Medical Feasibility").

   (2) A Means-Related Approach to Ordinary/Extraordinary Means.

   (3) The Projected Quality of the Patient's Life.

   (4) A Socially-Weighted Benefit/Burden Calculus.

In each instance the operative components are benefit, burden, patient's best interest, and social factors. How these are defined, prioritized, and "incorporated in" or "excluded from" the ethical question constitutes the ethical distinctions among them. Each of the succeeding chapters will deal with one of the four proposed **types**.

Each chapter will in some sense be a self-contained unit. The writings of a number of pertinent scholars will be brought together synthetically to illustrate the nontreatment standard proposed. Case applications will follow to demonstrate how the standard operates in practice. Each chapter will conclude with an analysis and critique of the major strengths and weaknesses of the proposed position. Finally, in a concluding chapter, this author's own position, culled and refined from the critique sections, will be set forth, destined to take its place among the others along the spectrum, open to rebuttal and further refinement.

In summary, then, this book represents a long search, a systematic survey and critique of the treatment/nontreatment literature related to handicapped newborns. Given the polarization and even sloganeering that frequently goes on between the various "schools of thought" represented here, it is hoped that the proposed four-option typology may serve as an analytical tool, a helpful framework to foster civil discourse and clarifying argument among advocates of opposing ethical viewpoints. Structuring the volume around these ethical models or types, the fundamental question remains ON WHAT BASIS IS THE DECISION TO FOREGO OR CEASE TREATMENT MADE?

NOTES

[1]President's Commission for the Study of Ethical Problems in Medicine and Bioethical and Behavioral Research, **Deciding**

to Forego Life-Sustaining Treatment (Washington, D.C.: U.S. Government Printing Office, 1983), pp. 197–207.

[2]Richard L. Lyons, "Physical and Mental Disabilities in Newborns Doubled in 25 Years," **New York Times** (18 July 1983), pp. 1, 10.

[3]Robin Marantz Henig and Anne B. Fletcher, "The Legacy of Prematurity," in **Your Premature Baby** (New York: Rawson Associates, 1983), pp. 224–231.

[4]"U.S. Population Up 2 Million," **The Washington Post** (1 January 1985). The 148,000 is derived by applying the 4% annual statistic of handicapped newborns to the total U.S. census statistic for infants born in 1984—3.7 million.

[5]David W. Smith, ed., **Recognizable Patterns of Human Malformation,** 2d ed. (Philadelphia: W.B. Saunders, 1976). Some helpful sources for medical data concerning "birth defects" include Robert Weir, **Selective Nontreatment of Handicapped Newborns** (New York: Oxford University Press, 1984), pp. 38–49; Robin Marantz Henig and Anne B. Fletcher, **Your Premature Baby,** pp. 63–97, 242–253; Gordon Avery, ed., **Neonatology: Pathophysiology and Management of the Newborn,** 2d ed. (Philadelphia: J.B. Lippincott Co., 1981); Richard E. Behrman and Victor C. Vaughan, eds., **Nelson's Textbook Pediatrics,** 12th ed. (Philadelphia: W.B. Saunders, 1983); Alexander Schaffer and Mary Ellen Avery, eds., **Diseases of Newborns,** 4th ed. (Philadelphia: W.B. Saunders, 1977).

[6]**Who Shall Survive?** Film produced by the Joseph P. Kennedy, Jr. Foundation, 1972.

[7]"Infant Died of Defects," **Bloomington Herald-Telephone,** 20 April 1982, p. 1; Joseph W. Rebone, " 'Minimal Quality of Life': Why Parents, Courts Choose Infant Doe's Death," **Hospital Progress** 63 (June 1982), pp. 10–14; In the

case of Bloomington's Infant Doe, the child's digestive blockage was a Traecheo-esophageal fistula in the throat, rather than a Duodenal atresia (Hopkins case), but the basic ethical problem and surgical correctability are the same for the two cases.

[8]Betty Lou Dotson, Director, Office of Civil Rights of the U.S. Department of Health and Human Services, "Notice to Health Care Providers," **Federal Register** 47 (June 16, 1982), p. 26027. Department of Health and Human Services Secretary Richard Schweiker had made the notice public on May 18, 1982. This ruling was conceived as an interpretation of Section 504 of the Rehabilitation Act (1973); First revision including Proposed Rules: Office of the Secretary, DHHS, "Nondiscrimination on the Basis of Handicap Relating to Health Care for Handicapped Infants," **Federal Register** 48 (July 5, 1983), pp. 30846–30852; Second revision: Office of the Secretary, DHHS, "Nondiscrimination on the Basis of Handicap Relating to Health Care for Handicapped Infants," **Federal Register** (January 12, 1984), pp. 1622–1654; Actual statute change: Child Abuse Amendments of 1984 [Public Law 98-457] (October 9, 1984); Proposed Regulations to implement statute change: Office of Human Development and Services, Department of Health and Human Services, "Child Abuse and Neglect Prevention and Treatment Program," **Federal Register** 49 (December 10, 1984), pp. 48160–48173; "Final Rule and Model Guidelines for Health Care Providers To Establish Infant Care Review Committees," **Federal Register** 50 (April 15, 1985), pp. 14878–14901. For a helpful evaluative survey of this entire legal process see Lawrence Brown, "Civil Rights and Regulatory Wrongs: The Reagan Administration and the Medical Treatment of Handicapped Infants," in **Journal of Health Politics, Policy and Law** 11 (Summer 1986), pp. 231–254.

[9]The Steinhaus Case was reported regularly in front page

stories by Robert Franklin in the **Minneapolis Star and Tribune** (8/22/86, 9/25/86, 10/15/86, 10/24/86, 10/27/86, 2/11/87).

[10]Erica M. Bates, "The Implications of Semantics of Developments in Medical Technology: The Fatal Consequence of Semantic Ignorance," **Et Cetera** 37 (Spring 1980), pp. 5–12.

[11]President's Commission, **Deciding to Forego,** Cover Letter, p. 5; For an historical study of parental/guardian rights see Earl Shelp, **Born to Die?** (New York: The Free Press, 1986), pp. 26–76.

[12]Some key resources on the ethics of Infanticide are Dennis Horan and Melinda Delahoyde, eds., **Infanticide and the Handicapped Newborn** (Provo: Brigham Young University, 1982); Marvin Kohl, ed., **Infanticide and the Value of Life** (Buffalo: Prometheus Books, 1978); Robert Weir, **Selective Nontreatment of Handicapped Newborns** (New York: Oxford University Press, 1984).

[13]Some of the key sources dealing with the "feeding" question are George Annas, "Nonfeeding: Lawful Killing in CA., Homicide in N.J.," **Hastings Center Report** 12 (December 1983), pp. 19–20; Daniel Callahan, "On Feeding the Dying," **Hastings Center Report** 13 (October 1983), p. 22; Alexander Morgan Capron, "Ironies and Tensions in Feeding the Dying," **Hastings Center Report** 13 (October 1984), pp. 32–35; Joanne Lynn, M.D. and James Childress, "Must Patients Always Be Given Food and Water?" **Hastings Center Report** 13 (October 1983), pp. 17–21; Richard A. McCormick, "Caring or Starving? The Case of Claire Conroy," **America** 152 (April 6, 1985), pp. 269–273; Gilbert Meilaender, "On Removing Food and Water: Against the Stream," **Hastings Center Report** 14 (December 1984), pp. 11–13; John J. Paris and Anne B. Fletcher, M.D., "Infant Doe Regulations and the Absolute Requirement to Use

Nourishment and Fluids For the Dying Infant," **Law, Medicine & Health Care** 11 (October 1983), pp. 210–213; Joanne Lynn, ed. **By No Extraordinary Means** (Bloomington: Indiana University Press, 1986).

[14]Charles E. Curran, "The Difference Between Personal Morality and Public Policy," in **Toward an American Catholic Moral Tradition** (Notre Dame: University of Notre Dame Press, 1987), pp. 194–202.

[15]One might begin a study of the legal questions surrounding nontreatment with the President's Commission, **Deciding to Forego.** Among the scholars who treat the legal questions surrounding handicapped newborns, the various articles of John A. Robertson are frequently cited. Here is a partial listing for further study: John A. Robertson, "Involuntary Euthanasia of Defective Newborns: A Legal Analysis," **Stanford Law Review** 27 (1975), pp. 213–269; Robertson and Norman Fost, "Passive Euthanasia of Defective Newborn Infants: Legal Considerations," **Journal of Pediatrics** 88 (May 1976), pp. 883–889; Robertson, "Discretionary Nontreatment of Defective Newborns," in **Genetics and the Law,** eds. Aubrey Milunsky and George Annas (New York: Plenum Press, 1976), pp. 451–465; Robertson, "Legal Issues in Nontreatment of Defective Newborns," in **Decision-making and the Defective Newborn,** ed. Chester Swinyard, pp. 359–383.

[16]David Karnofsky, **Time** (3 November 1961), p. 60.

[17]Joseph Fletcher, **Humanhood: Essays in Biomedical Ethics** (Buffalo: Prometheus Books, 1979), p. 150; See also Daniel C. Maguire, **Death by Choice** (New York: Doubleday & Co./Schocken Paperback, 1973, 1974), pp. 122–123; Paul Ramsey, **The Patient as Person: Explorations in Medical Ethics** (New Haven: Yale University Press, 1970), pp. 147–148; David

Karnofsky, "Why Prolong the Life of a Patient with Advanced Cancer?" **Cancer Journal of Clinicians** 10 (January–February 1960), pp. 10ff.

[18]Notre Dame theologian James T. Burtchaell wrote such an impassioned critique of an article by Paul Johnson, which appeared in the **Linacre Quarterly**. This strong defense of the right of every child to life borders on a vitalistic mandate, though he never states so as such. See James T. Burtchaell, "How Much Should a Child Cost? A Response to Paul Johnson," **Linacre Quarterly** 47 (February 1980), pp. 54–63; see also James T. Burtchaell, "How Much Is a Child Worth? From Abortion to Infanticide," in **Rachel Weeping and Other Essays on Abortion** (Kansas City: Andrews and McMeel, 1982), pp. 288–320.

Chapter One

A Medical Indications Policy

> A medical indications policy is the only way to take a middle
> path between relentless treatment of the voiceless dying,
> which refuses to let them die even when disease or injury has
> won, and killing or hastening death or neglecting to sustain
> those who simply are voiceless incurables. The latter has to
> date been deemed to be manslaughter in some degree. Mor-
> ally, it is never right to turn against the good of human life.
> In the case of one's own life, public policy could go so far as
> to place that in an area of liberties. But to allow private in-
> dividuals to turn against the good of **another's** life would be
> to promote injustice (P. Ramsey **Ethics at the Edges of Life,**
> p. 188).

On February 9, 1974, a handicapped son was born to Lor-
raine and Robert Houle of Portland, Maine. Baby Boy Houle's
birth defects included "the absence of a left eye, a rudimentary
left ear with no ear canal, a malformed left thumb and a tracheal
esophageal fistula."[1] Further medical evaluation indicated the
lack of response of the infant's right eye to light stimuli, the presence of some non-fused vertebrae, and the "virtual certainty" of
some anoxia-related brain damage. In order to allow for normal
digestion and respiration, relatively immediate surgery would be

required to remove the tracheal esophageal fistula. The parents decided to withhold consent for the procedure. Pediatrician Martin A. Barron, Jr., and the Maine Medical Center filed suit in Cumberland County Superior Court, seeking to override the parents' decision and to secure Court permission to perform the "life-saving" surgery. Despite efforts to stabilize and maintain the infant during this brief flurry of legal proceedings, Baby Boy Houle's condition deteriorated. Periods of apnea (intermittent breath stoppages), pneumonia, and convulsive seizures were treated with artificial devices and appropriate medications. On February 14, Justice David Roberts ruled:

> . . . at the moment of live birth there does exist a human being entitled to the fullest protection of the law. The most basic right enjoyed by every human being is the right to life itself.

> . . . Were it his [the physician's] opinion that life itself could not be preserved, heroic measures ought not be required. However, the doctor's qualitative evaluation of the value of the life to be preserved is not legally within the scope of his expertise.

> In the court's opinion the issue before the court is not the prospective quality of the life to be preserved, but the medical feasibility of the proposed treatment compared with the almost certain risk of death should treatment be withheld. Being satisfied that corrective surgery is medically necessary and medically feasible, the court finds that the defendants herein have no right to withhold such treatment and that to do so constitutes neglect in the legal sense.[2]

Despite the subsequent surgery and intensive therapeutic care, Baby Boy Houle died on February 24, at the age of fifteen days.

Maine Superior Court Justice Roberts exemplifies well the so-called "medical indications" or "medical feasibility" policy to be surveyed and critiqued in this chapter. Eschewing any utilitarian measurement of human potential or projections of acceptable versus unacceptable qualities of life, advocates of the "medical indications" standard hold high the banner of the inherent equality of all human beings. In their estimation, access to society's health care facilities and resources ought to be based solely on biological need. Thus, as Justice Roberts noted, if a treatment or surgical procedure is "medically necessary and medically feasible," i.e., physiologically beneficial, it is thereby morally obligatory. Some leeway in public policy might be allowed for a competent patient to interpret "benefit" for oneself and thus refuse a debatable or risky procedure. However, ethically-speaking, for competent patients as well as for the voiceless non-competent, what is medically beneficial ought to be morally obligatory.[3]

A thorough search of the literature yields two scholars, Christian ethicist Paul Ramsey and public policy expert Elizabeth MacMillan, who develop a "medical indications" or a "medical feasibility" policy at any depth.[4] Other scholars gathered under this rubric generally affirm Ramsey's efforts (Sherlock, Dyck, and Meilaender) or MacMillan's legal analysis (Soskin, Vitello). Civil rights coalitions and conservative public policy advocates also gravitate toward a "medical indications" policy as the tightest ethical and legal safeguard against the abuse of handicapped citizens.[5] Likewise, the controversial 1982 "Baby Doe Rule" of the Department of Health and Human Services and its subsequent revisions reflect a "medical indications" approach to neonatal nontreatment decisions.[6] Finally, a number of practicing physicians, most notably Surgeon General C. Everett Koop and Eugene Diamond, seem to adopt this position, though their writings are frequently more medical and homiletic than strictly ethical.

This chapter will be divided into four sections. The first section will examine the fundamental presuppositions that undergird a medical indications approach to nontreatment decisions. Then we will briefly look at four alternative treatment standards from the critical vantage point of medical indications policy proponents. Accepting, for the moment, Ramsey's rejection of these standards as ethically inadequate, the next section will present a full account of a medical indications policy. What is a **medical indications** policy? How does it apply to the cases of handicapped infants? For which cases of "defective" newborns is treatment medically and thereby morally indicated? In what circumstances is treatment medically infeasible and morally contra-indicated? Of particular interest will be the non-terminal cases where the patient is judged to be "marginally alive" or maintaining only "insensate existence." Finally, the chapter will conclude with a critique of the medical indications standard.

Fundamental Presuppositions and Methodology

Behind Judge Roberts' ruling, as behind the various presentations of a medical indications policy to be synthesized and surveyed here, are several fundamental assumptions. Whether rooted in specifically Christian religious beliefs about creation or grounded in some philosophical theory of human nature, rights, and widely held societal values, all proponents of a medical indications policy affirm the following presuppositions:

(1) the inherent dignity of every human life;

(2) the radical equality of all human life;

(3) responsible persons have interrelational obligations one to another;

(4) a heavily deontological (law-based, absolutistic) ethic.

1. The **inherent dignity** (or sanctity) **of every human life**, regardless of handicaps or developmental potential, will be a cornerstone principle for three of the four "types" to be surveyed in this volume. The Judaeo-Christian tradition regards every human life, even those severely deformed, as sacred from

the moment of birth (or even conception) to the grave. "Sacred," or hallowed, refers not only to a belief in the divine origin of all human life, but also to the faith assertion that each human being, irrespective of functional handicaps, is fashioned in the image and likeness of the Holy One, God the Creator (Gen 1:27; 5:1–3). For Protestant ethicist Paul Ramsey, this sanctity of each individual is rooted in a Barthian sense of "holy awe" and "respect" for human "life as a divine loan." Ramsey sees this abiding dignity as "alien," a gift which humans neither earn nor relinquish. Speaking of his neighbor as "holy ground," Ramsey believes that "an individual human life is absolutely unique, inviolable, irreplaceable, noninterchangeable, not substitutable, and not meldable with other lives. . . ."[7]

Nor is knowledge of the inherent value of all human life restricted to Judaeo-Christian believers. Natural reason can extrapolate human dignity from the fundamental instinct of self-preservation.[8] Anyone advocating respect for all living things would also necessarily adopt this corollary of respect for all **human** living things. Philosophers, like John Rawls and William Frankena, base their equality theories of justice on some rational presumption of intrinsic human worth and rights. So also, the American legal principle of equal protection of the law rests on a respect life premise. The world community has assented to this core value in the United Nations' **International Bill of Human Rights.**

> . . . recognition of the inherent dignity and of the equal and inalienable rights of all members of the human family is the foundation of freedom, justice, and peace in the world.[9]

Ramsey strengthens this emphasis on the abiding worth of every living human being by affirming that human life is embodied life, that man is "a sacredness in the natural biological order."[10] Any dualistic separation of one's so-called "spiritual" or rational nature from one's biological existence is categorically rejected. Every living human is not only a being of moral worth in the social and political order, but a value in and of oneself—an "embodied soul" or an "ensouled body"—a person. Such body-soul unity leads medical indications proponents to a strong preference for the preservation of biological life as a defense against any decision which smacks of otherworldly asceticism or of a functional definition of "person." Biological life or physiological functioning is viewed as a constitutive component of the value of human life, not an instrumental or directly expendable good.

This strong emphasis on "embodied life" leads Ramsey to see the refusal of potentially life-saving procedures as a rejection of the value of life itself, a choice for death. If "(t)he conviction that one should always choose life lies at the heart of the practice of medicine and nursing," then to choose death, either directly as an end or by foregoing beneficial, life-saving treatment "is to throw the gift back in the face of the giver."[11] Utah State University scholar Richard Sherlock summarizes this physiologically-oriented "pro-life" presumption in a general principle that he believes to be self-evident and non-controversial.

> Where it is possible to do so, and especially as it involves one's professional responsibilities, one should choose to save those lives that one is capable of saving.[12]

2. A second fundamental presupposition of the medical indications typology is in some sense a corollary of the dignity of life principle—the radical equality of all human life. The inherent worth or dignity of life itself, even with the corresponding right to life guarantee, is in itself no defense against the judgment that some lives are worth more/less than others. In triage situations involving scarce resources or even in the ordinary distribution of available medical care, one could respectfully prior-

itize patients according to some amalgamation of human qualities (often personal and social over against biological), relegating those patients deemed "lesser" or "substandard" to the end of the treatment line. Proponents of a medical indications policy see such quality of life judgments in the normal course of neonatal medicine as inherently discriminatory and ethically unjust. The "naked equality of one life with another" is THE benchmark of a medical indications approach to treatment decisions.[13] The corresponding human and civil right is obvious— **the equal right of all to medical treatment,** with some presumed obligation on society to provide such resources and care.

Human rights advocates are particularly fearful of societal bias against the handicapped, based on some quality of life projection for "perfect life" over against "deformed existence."[14] Passage of the Rehabilitation Act by the United States Congress in 1973 enshrined in law this moral right of each and all to equal access to society's health care resources and facilities, regardless of handicaps or functional potential. Medical indications proponents believe that one's handicap or deformity as such ought not be the basis for deciding to treat or withhold therapy from a living, embodied, and therefore de facto "worthy" human patient.

Attorney Ronald Soskin and Rutgers professor S. John Vitello together summarized the above presuppositions succinctly regarding handicapped newborns:

> The basic position is that by providing care for defective newborns, society's commitment to the values of life and equality are reinforced, producing respect for the life and moral equality of all persons. The proposition is fundamental—human life must be protected "for its own sake because it is what it is," and because "it is vitally necessary for the law to maintain the salutary principle that all human life is within its protection."[15]

In short, Ramsey reflects well the dignity and equality of life presuppositions of the medical indications stance in asserting that therapeutic, palliative, and humane medical "care" cannot and ought not fall short of universal equality.[16]

3. A third presupposition focuses on the conviction that **reasonable, responsible persons have some interrelational obligations to one another** and to the commonweal. As children of God, or merely as rational members of the species, we are each responsible not only for our personal welfare, but also to some extent for the well-being of others, particularly those entrusted to us or for whom we have accepted responsibility. Thus, spouses or covenanted friends are presumed to be responsible one for another. Parents, teachers, and governments are assumed to be obligated to and for their offspring, students, and the citizenry respectively. What Ramsey calls in a religious context "covenant fidelity" and "canons of loyalty" can, to a large extent, be equated with "partnerships," "contracts," and the "strings attached" to all commitments in human relationships, both those which precede choice and those which are contingent upon it.[17] A society is obliged to protect the dignity and equality of all its members, with a special watchfulness on behalf of "the weak and the helpless"—children, the mentally incompetent, and minorities in general.[18]

The art of medicine, as one arena of human relational interdependence, calls for health care professionals (especially the physician) and the competent patient to join together as co-adventurers in search of healing and comfort for the patient. The physician is neither almighty parent nor subservient employee. So also, the competent patient is neither an autonomous health care consumer nor a "voiceless" object. Both patient and physician are bonded together in the common search for a cure, for palliative comfort, and for a return to the fullest level of mental and physical functioning possible, given one's age, condition, and prognostic potential.

Medical indications advocates agree, therefore, that "the patient's best interest" is and ought to be the focus of this joint medical venture. A corollary to this is the presumption that to decide one's best interest "for" a competent patient without his/her participation and consent would be to reduce that patient to an **object,** which can never be in that patient's best interest. In the cases of non-competent patients, such as all handicapped infants, focusing exclusively on the child's best interests as a basis for decision making forestalls the potential familial and social bias that may creep into "substituted judgments" or a so-called "reasonable person" standard.

It should be noted early on that medical indications policy advocates tend to interpret a given patient's "best interest" quite narrowly, that is, more individualistically and more physiologically than even the relatively strict ordinary/extraordinary means advocates would do. Attempts to incorporate familial or social burdens, even those which might impinge on a patient's own psychological sense of well-being, are suspect as omens of a creeping quality of life bias against a given patient's absolute right to life and its protection. To prevent possible injustice against a non-competent patient's best interest by an erroneous or selfish proxy judgment, medical indications proponents seek both to restrict parental and guardian autonomy and to define a patient's best interest as objectively and narrowly as possible.

4. If the philosophical term "deontology" is defined accurately as an ethical method which exclusively, or at least heavily, stresses duty and fidelity to one's obligations, then **a medical indications policy is** foursquare **a deontological ethic.** Fearful of teleological ethics—based on future potential or utility—as threatening to the inherent values, equal rights, and corresponding duties noted above, advocates of a medical indications policy agree that "a deontological dimension or test holds chief place in medical ethics, beside teleological considerations."[19]

Paul Ramsey has consistently advocated an ethic of obediential response to the unconditional demands of agape or covenant fidelity.[20] Whether spoken of in such specifically religious language or described more generically as an ethic of obligation to our avowed and ex officio commitments, a medical indications policy gives first priority to duty in the name of the respect owed to the equal dignity of each and all. The fundamental presuppositions and rights noted above lay duty claims on competent patients, parents, physicians, and society that are prior to and independent of any calculus of net utility or qualitative benefit. The consequential **goal** sought ought never negate the abiding dignity and rights posited here.

While avowedly anti-utilitarian, medical indications advocates are not thereby pure deontologists. Their willingness to incorporate consequences into the ethical enterprise, albeit secondarily and primarily in situations where "the disease has won," indicates some variation on the "mixed deontology" or "moderate teleology" methodologies as coined by Curran, McCormick, Frankena, May, and others.[21] However, a medical indications approach to decision making is predominantly and admittedly a more duty-oriented and absolutist schema than any of the other types to be surveyed here. Fidelity to the fundamental presuppositions cited above holds sway against any potential or net benefit. Only when life-saving becomes a non-option can medical indications proponents arguably be said to shift to a consequential weighing of prospective qualities of life related to the brief meantime called the dying process.

In summary, a medical indications policy rests on the inherent dignity and equality of **every** human life, incarnated in human covenants or binding relationships, both those freely chosen and those which precede and ground human election. It is the absolute, incontrovertible duty of society, health care professionals, parents or guardians, and competent patients "to preserve, protect, and defend" the right of all patients to life and to equitable medical treatment. The right to life, interpreted in terms of an inextricably conjoined body-soul unity, is given substance in the ethical mandate to always choose life. If independent biological functioning can be sustained, that is without merely being permanently attached to artificial life support equipment, then one ought to choose such life, irrespective of one's qualitative potential. Medical indications proponents define "life" and "patient's best interest" primarily in physiological terms, lest non-medical qualities of life threaten this human body-soul unity, relegating the biological dimension of life to secondary, instrumental, and expendable status.

"Name the Enemy"—
A Critique of Inadequate Standards

Rarely if ever do ethicists create pristine theories in a vacuum. Advocacy of a "medical indications" approach to decisions emerges both in ethics and in public policy debates as a solution, a viable alternative to decision making standards judged inadequate or even unjust. In **Ethics at the Edges of Life,** Ramsey lists five possible policies or standards "for when and how medical care should be extended or when it should be withheld or withdrawn":

(1) a standard-medical-care policy;

(2) a patient's right to refuse treatment;

(3) a quality-of-expected-life policy;

(4) the ordinary/extraordinary distinction;

(5) a medical indications policy.[22]

He quickly rejects the first two of these as wholly inadequate. On the more abstract or objective end of the spectrum, reducing all treatment decisions to "a standard-medical-care policy," as if the emphasis is primarily on the availability or "ordinariness" of the means qua means, is to do a disservice to the **patient's** best interest (diagnosis, prognosis, and relative situation), which ought to be the central focus of all medico-moral decisions. The usualness, availability, and generic usefulness of given means comprise only one component of the ethical equation.

On the opposite, more subjective end of the spectrum, reducing the ultimate interpretation of burdens, benefits, and options to a patient's right to refuse any or all treatment tends too facilely to baptize the autonomy principle. If a patient is competent s/he has a right and duty to participate in the decision making process. However, such a right is not to be confused with libertine autonomy. A patient is free to contribute to the debate of what will benefit him or her, but ultimately, morally-speaking, s/he is not arbitrarily free to refuse reasonably beneficial measures. A patient's freedom and dignity do not encompass the right to do wrong, nor a right to assault the value of one's own life by refusing objectively therapeutic treatment. "Treatments are not electable because elected, desirable because desired."[23]

In a somewhat tangential treatment of Robert Veatch's "so-called reasonable man standard," Ramsey criticizes Veatch's adoption of the "patient's perspective" as an illustration of excessive autonomy infringing on objective moral duty.[24] **Reasonableness**, like **patient's best interest**, is a nebulous or formal concept. If one defines the "reasonable" course of action as that which is medically indicated or morally binding, then Ramsey has no major objections to a reasonable person standard. However, when "reasonable" is wedded to an absolute license on the patient's part to decide what constitutes the reasonable choice, then Ramsey sees subjectivism and voluntarism usurping the central role of duty and objectivity.

The potential for abuse is evident. Competent patients, or worse still the guardians of non-competents, would be free to accept or reject **any** treatment, irrespective of its potential medical benefit. Writing primarily from a public policy perspective,

Veatch asserts "that no competent patients have ever been forced to undergo any medical treatment for their own good no matter how misguided their refusal may have appeared."[25] While such a right to refuse treatment "for any reason" may be emerging in law, Ramsey rejects Veatch's claim that such autonomy is our **legal** heritage and asserts it ought not be our **ethical** future. Even if, as Ramsey hypothetically grants, such autonomy is condoned as a public policy safeguard of individual rights from tyranny by some central power, the absolute right of a patient to refuse any treatment as an ethical thesis wrongly baptizes subjectivism over objectivity, whim over duty, and license over canons of loyalty. Medical indications proponents fear that the adoption of "a patient's right to refuse treatment" as one's sole ethical criterion "moves too far in the direction of subjective voluntarism and automated physicians."[26]

Rejecting "a standard-medical-care policy" as too abstract and "a patient's right to refuse treatment" policy as potentially too subjective, Ramsey next challenges the incorporation of "quality-of-expected-life" elements into treatment decisions. Medical indications proponents level their harshest and most univocal criticism at all quality-of-expected-life standards.[27] Richard Sherlock, whose "general principle" mandating life-saving procedures whenever possible was cited earlier, accuses quality of life advocates of revising that principle with an unacceptable exception clause:

> When it is possible . . . one should save life except where the life saved will be a life that is not worth living anyway.[28]

Whether expressed in terms of "minimal" existence, absence of a "life worth living," or an "extraordinarily burdened" life, a quality of life standard bases medical treatment decisions in the present on some prediction of the type of life this patient will live post-treatment. If the prognosis is for an extremely poor standard of living, whatever elements one incorporates into determining "poor," then that life is "a life not worth living." The patient, it is presumed, would be "better off dead" or, at least, better off dying sooner than later.

Medical indications proponents worry about the inherent vagueness and imprecision of establishing that line of demarcation between an acceptable and an unbearable quality of life. For them the primary problem with the quality of life standard is the difficulty of applying it in any consistent manner to yield predictable results. They believe that quality of life determinations involve several factors, none of which can be defined or measured with enough accuracy to avoid arbitrary, ad hoc decisions. Such a standard lends itself to bias, incquities, and injustice. More importantly, because a quality of life standard assumes that some lives are not worth saving, it "undermines widely held social values."[29] Ramsey denounces all such attempts to base treatment decisions on some hypothetical standard for "meaningful life" as a violation of the basic human covenants of care and a fundamental injustice against the inherent equal and alien dignity of every human being.[30] It is the potential "slippery slope" that most frightens medical indications proponents. Once any list of qualities of expected life, however reasonable and/or restricted, is allowed to impinge on the absolute right of **all** patients, regardless of handicaps, to equal medical treatment, the slope to an unjust caste system, and eventually to involuntary euthanasia, is paved and greased.

The final medical policy that Ramsey critiques is the distinction between ordinary and extraordinary means, viewed as synonyms for "imperative" versus "electable or morally dispensable" treatments respectively. He is somewhat reluctant to jettison the concepts comprising the ordinary/extraordinary means standard, even if the language has been used ambiguously. The terms **ordinary** and **extraordinary**, "however cumbersome, opaque, and unilluminating," directed attention to objective consideration both of the patient's condition and of "the armamentarium of medicine's remedies." As Ramsey interprets the ordinary/extraordinary means tradition, it was and is an attempt to steer an objective midcourse between an abstract, descriptive classification of means qua means on the one hand and a purely arbitrary and subjective canonization of a patient's wishes on the other.[31]

While applauding this quest for objectivity, its patient-centeredness, and the rationale for not prolonging dying with useless means, Ramsey ultimately comes face to face with the unmistakable quality of life elements that the ordinary/extraordinary means tradition factors into the cases of patients not irreversibly dying. Linking those projected qualities to **causation by means,** as contemporary ordinary/extraordinary means advocates do, does nothing to forestall the medical indications proponents' objections against any standard that bases treatment decisions in the present on some judgment about the quality or "livability" of **future** existence post-treatment. Grateful to the ordinary/extraordinary means tradition for attempting an **objective** synthesis of the various ethical components—availability of means, prognosis for given patients, and degree of related burdens—and yet fearful of the inherent quality-of-expected-life elements in all decisions to withhold medically beneficial or life-saving treatment from patients not irretrievably dying, Ramsey prefaces his own presentation of a medical indications policy by stating:

> Perhaps it could be said that a medical indications policy is a more subtle and more patient-oriented modulation of what is meant by ordinary/extraordinary and the customary medical practice standards. Perhaps a medical indications policy is the growing edge of those summaries. . . . I shall argue that the significant moral meaning of these similar and related standards can be reduced almost without significant remainder to a medical indications policy.[32]

A "Medical Indications Policy" and Handicapped Newborns

Ramsey's reluctance to let go of the ordinary/extraordinary means standard rests primarily on his similar desire for a policy that is somehow objective as well as related to each patient's condition. In **The Patient as Person** Ramsey came to grips with level one of what he later calls "a medical indications policy"— **the cases of irreversibly dying patients**, both competent and non-competent. For Ramsey "dying" is synonymous with **irreversibly** or **imminently** dying. Thus, the often cited Johns Hopkins Baby (Down's Syndrome with duodenal atresia), who might be said to be dying if the duodenal atresia were not removed, is, in Ramsey's categories, not dying because his life, that is, a prolongation of biological functioning not maintained by auxiliary equipment, is salvageable. Restricting the term **dying** only to those patients irreversibly at death's door offers Ramsey a seemingly clear-cut physiological line of demarcation. However, it lends itself to some confusion in dialogue with others who define "dying" more broadly in terms of a life-threatening condition, which, if not removed, will cause death.

Ramsey's core medical indications thesis is this: If a patient, competent or otherwise, has entered the dying process, in which all curative efforts are futile or at best serve only minimally to forestall the **imminently** inevitable, then such medical procedures are optional, perhaps even contra-indicated.[33] The conscious, competent, irreversibly dying patient may choose to continue curative efforts, such as experimental drugs or risky procedures, in the faint hope of a "miraculous" victory over death, provided availability, cost, and deprivation of another do not override the probable futility of such extraordinary measures. If nothing else, such heroic efforts may comfort the patient and family with the knowledge that they did all they could to save her/him. However, the conscious, competent irreversibly dying patient may also morally choose to forego such relatively useless efforts in order to die more peacefully or humanely, surrounded by the supportive "care" of kith and kin. Neither option contradicts Ramsey's categorical imperative, "never abandon care." The only exception to the right of competent irreversibly dying patients to refuse such minimally beneficial treatment would be if some special duty, "such as affording them an opportunity to make a will or to have their last reconciliation with God or a family member," required a brief prolongation of life.[34] Admitting his own inability to determine when, in fact, the "process of dying" has irreversibly taken hold, Ramsey bows to medical science.

> The reply must be that this is a medical judgment and that physicians can and do determine—in human, no doubt fallible judgment—the difference between dying and nondying terminal patients. In the case of those whose death is impending, further attempted salvic treatment can only prolong dying.[35]

In the case of **non-competent** irreversibly dying patients, particularly infants or the severely mentally impaired who are voiceless, the patient's best interest, medically-speaking, is to be the focus of the decision. If treatment is practically useless or only of psychological comfort with no appreciable physiological benefit, then a parent or guardian or someone ought to be free either to consent to these extraordinary efforts or to shift toward (only) caring for the dying patient.

Both Ramsey and MacMillan place the decision making locus "in between" the physician and parents. The role of the physician is primary and vital, but still a limited one. Only s/he can more or less objectively match proposed means with a given patient's condition to project potential medical benefit or futility. If the patient is irreversibly dying and all medical treatment will serve **only** to prolong that dying process, then the physician rightly steps back and parents are the ordinary locus for deciding whether to continue relatively useless efforts or whether to shift over to hospice-like care for the dying. Courts enter the decision making arena as a last resort only if parental or medical neglect is suspected.[36] Ramsey says very little on the question of a parental decision to continue aggressive, albeit futile efforts if they so choose. The law tends to allow such "excess," though limited resources and a medical judgment of **absolute** uselessness may be brought to bear. Generally, the infant takes the matter to a "Higher Court" soon enough that parental wishes to prolong relatively useless treatment are respected as psychologically therapeutic for the mourners while not categorically inconsistent with the infant's best interests.[37]

The only neonatal illustration of a patient born irreversibly dying cited by Ramsey is the "anencephalic baby," whose lack of the upper or frontal lobes of the brain indicates reasonably imminent death with no option for reversal. Ramsey also toys with defining such anencephalic newborns as not being born alive. This "curious exception" will be taken up later in this chapter. Elizabeth MacMillan mentions infants with Trisomy 13 or Trisomy 18 as examples of patients born already dying. The presence of a third chromosome at the thirteenth or eighteenth pairing causes severe, unalterable mental deformity. At most death could be forestalled only for a few extra "unresponsive" months through aggressive, costly, but ultimately useless means. By contrast, Ramsey mentions a Tay-Sachs baby as an example of a non-dying terminal case. Such an infant "is destined to die," and will, within the first few years of life, be seized irretrievably by the dying process, but ought not be judged so at birth, "presymptomatically."

Therefore, a medical indications policy acknowledges the right of imminently, irreversibly dying patients **or their guardians** to accept or forego heroic, relatively useless means. The decision of how to live while dying—betubed and fighting all the way or in a more hospice-like setting, relatively free of medical apparatus—requires qualitative judgments, open to a breadth of interpretation, once the question of life-saving itself has exceeded human grasp. However, the fact that irreversibly dying patients are not obliged to accept further useless curative efforts "ought not to be carelessly applied to the case of defective newborns."[38] Being born handicapped, even severely so, and/or with a correctable life-threatening condition signifies a "need for help," **not** a license for abandonment nor a false relegation to the category "dying."

In the cases of patients, competent or non-competent, **who are not irreversibly dying,** a medical indications policy asserts that any treatment that prognostically will be medically beneficial is automatically morally indicated. Comparing various treatment options or the medical benefit of treatment versus nontreatment keeps the decision more objective, more physiological or scientific, and thus more focused on what is "medically indicated," rather than prejudicially judging whose life is worth saving.

Ramsey speaks directly to the so-called "wretched" cases, where the prognosis is tragic or far from ideal, but in which the patient is not (yet) in the throes of dying.

> Where a prognosis of fatal illness, severe uncorrectable defect, incurability, or nonrecovery has been made in the case of voiceless nondying patients, there will be some cases in which purely medical interventions will serve to improve patients' conditions of life, others in which nothing helps. In either case, there remains an undiminished obligation first of all to sustain life and, in the second instance, to use palliative treatments where possible.[39]

The phrase "conditions of life" might be seen as indicating some quality-of-expected-life determination, but Ramsey counters that improvement of one's biological functioning and physiological capabilities still remains in the objective realm of medical benefit. The medical venture is focused not only on saving life, but at restoring one to the fullest physiological functioning possible within one's finite limitations. "Good health" is **better** than mere "survival," even though that survival is presumed to be a life worth living, or at least a life one ought never declare not worth living.

Therefore, in the vast majority of the so-called "Baby Doe" Cases, Ramsey and his medical indications associates would decide in favor of treatment. Mentally handicapped infants (frequently with Down's Syndrome) ought not be declared "dying" and allowed to do so just because some reversible life-threatening anomaly presently inhibits normal food digestion. Surgery to correct the esophageal fistula or the duodenal atresia is medically feasible, biologically beneficial, and therefore ought to be morally obligatory. What can be done to save life and to promote a modicum of good or improved health ought to be done. In Ramsey's perspective, to refuse such life-saving treatment is tantamount to killing the infant, choosing death over life, albeit by indirect causation.

To further nuance terms like "medical," "benefit," "futile," and "useless," Ramsey states firmly that "medical criteria for care should remain physiological."

> The tests for telling whether to discontinue treatments should be clinical or physiological ones (if these are the proper words for my meaning), not anyone's "values." They should not **in themselves**, with or without intention, build into the conditions for allowing the dying to die a discriminatory definition of a life worth living.[40]

Restricting the arena of the medical enterprise to physiological or biological concerns forestalls the potential injustice inevitable, according to Ramsey, if medical practitioners begin determining access to treatment based on their own socio-economic-religious trans-biological values.

Ramsey singles out the eminent pediatric surgeon R. B. Zachary of Children's Hospital, Sheffield, England, as a paradigmatic medical indications policy practitioner.[41] A prime focus of Dr. Zachary's surgical practice and writing since 1948 has been the treatment of spina bifida babies. Approximately twice in every one thousand births in this country an infant is born with spina bifida cystica, literally an "open spine" with a "cyst" or a meningocele protruding through the opening. Depending on the condition of the neural fibers in the protruding sac, its location along the spine, and the feasibility of surgery to close the opening, the infant's prognosis varies from terminal to treatable, with varying degrees of disability. Since the neural tissue in this exposed area is abnormal, the muscles innervated by it will in most cases be partly or completely paralyzed. Lower limb movement as well as bladder and bowel control is frequently affected, requiring later surgeries and other long-term therapies. In addition, about 90% of all infants with myelomeningocele develop hydrocephalus. Implantation and subsequent replacement of shunt valves are thus often medically indicated. With proper care and medical watchfulness, most myelomeningocele children fall within the lower normal I.Q. range. Finally, the unopposed action of certain muscles can further curve the spine, a condition called kyphosis, which may require only partially beneficial corrective surgery.[42]

Zachary takes issue with his Sheffield colleague, Dr. John Lorber, who, in the late 1960s, shifted from prescribing aggressive treatment for the vast majority of spina bifida babies to a policy of selective nontreatment based on six medical factors, which Lorber believes are determinable in the first day of neonatal life.[43] Dr. Zachary protests both the validity of Lorber's criteria as well as the false impression that nontreatment means that the infant is somehow irreversibly in the process of dying. Not only is a myelomeningocele infant not usually irreversibly dying, but most often the open lesion, even if left untreated, is not a life-threatening condition in any immediate sense.

Zachary challenges the statistics set forth by proponents of selective nontreatment, who claim a high mortality rate, near 100%, for those infants left untreated. He makes it clear that the nursing care or "management" they receive is suspect at best. One pediatrician admits to prescribing 60 mg. per kg. of body weight of chloral hydrate, four times daily. **Nelson's Pediatrics** recommends 1/8 that dosage as a sedative and 1/4 that amount for hypnosis. Rejecting the assertion that such prescriptions are primarily palliative, Zachary accuses these pediatricians of deliberately doping those infants selected out, so that they will not request food (cry or suck) and will thereby waste away within a few days or weeks at most.[44] Zachary sees such subtle, "indirect" infanticide, as unjust, an "inbuilt insurance policy" against the survival of nontreated spina bifida patients.

By contrast, Zachary prescribes surgical closure of the lesion as medically feasible and indicated in **all but two instances.** The first category, perfectly in line with a medical indications policy, are those infants who are judged irreversibly terminal, for whom death is imminent within days, a week, or a little longer at most. The presence of massive intracranial hemorrhage, severe congenital heart disease, or another unalterable life-threatening anomaly supersedes any benefit normally to be derived from the otherwise indicated back surgery.

Zachary's second nontreatment category is a subset of those myelomeningocele infants who are seriously afflicted, but not terminal in any immediate sense. In these cases, Zachary's medical criterion is based on the size and condition of the lesion itself. If the lesion is too wide and/or the myelomeningocele is extremely large, or if it produces a severe spine curvature (kyphosis), the possibility of wound breakdown and serious infection is great. Surgery may well do more harm than good and is thus medically contra-indicated. Simple dressing and protection of the wound may better allow epithelium to naturally grow over the exposed area, which, while not an ideal "cure," is proportionately a better medical option for the infant than surgery.

The timing and degree of spinal surgery for all others will depend on the medical urgency of the case. If there are signs at birth of leg movement or some muscle activity in the hips, more immediate surgery will inhibit further loss. According to Zachary, all non-dying infants, whether their lesions are surgically treated or not, ought to be offered the proper therapeutic procedures for hydrocephalus, renal tract difficulties, and related orthopedic problems.

In Ramsey's estimation, Zachary's approach is a par excellence reflection of a medical indications policy. While acknowledging that Dr. Zachary finds himself in "broad agreement" with Richard McCormick's relational quality-of-life standard, Ramsey questions if in fact Zachary is really ever transcending the strictly physiological sphere in his nontreatment criteria.[45] Ramsey sees Zachary's proposals throughout as based solely on what is "medically good" for the patient—to reduce physiological handicaps to a minimum, to avoid infection or wound breakdown, and to preserve as much muscle and/or leg activity as possible. Zachary believes that his "fundamental purpose is not to add years to their lives but to add life to their years." Ramsey asserts that in each case Zachary's measurement of good/bad or of quality versus quantity of years is biologically-based, the maximum physiological functioning possible given one's limitations. If not irreversibly dying, the myelomeningocele infant deserves the best medical efforts available to enhance his/her participation in life, however brief or extended. For Ramsey this is a medical indications policy respectfully applied.

Harvard scholar Arthur Dyck adopts Ramsey's medical indications approach as "an excellent resolution of the debate" concerning "what would and should guide us in making medical decisions regarding handicapped newborns and incompetents generally."[46] Only if a patient is irreversibly dying or if one's medical situation is incurable is it moral to forego further (futile) therapies. Even in cases with very tragic circumstances, such as the irreparably comatose or the severely brain damaged (no functioning of the cerebral cortex), Dyck's ethic of benemortasia would strongly presume in favor of continued treatment "until there is no reasonable hope of improving or reversing the condition."

Ramsey's former student, ethicist Gilbert Meilaender, defends his mentor's medical indications policy as the "most attractive alternative"—"if not fully satisfactory in every case—a rule of practice which embodies genuine moral discernment."[47] However, Meilaender zeros in on a potential inequity, or at least inconsistency, in Ramsey's reluctance to categorically reject all quality-of-expected-life elements, particularly with reference to competent patients. Obviously, if a patient is imminently and irreversibly dying, that patient or one's caretakers may factor in quality of life judgments concerning how to live while dying. However, Meilaender also points out that Ramsey concedes that the quality-of-expected life (burden) element "in the meaning of the ordinary/extraordinary distinction . . . may still be a test applied by a patient competent to refuse medical treatment."[48] Although such a willingness to allow burden to outweigh potential medical benefit contradicts the basic thrust of the medical indications policy surveyed here, Meilaender rightly points out Ramsey's flirtations with allowing competent patients to include "morally relevant nonmedical factors" in deciding to forego treatment. If such inclusion were valid for competent patients, then Meilaender surmises that a medical indications policy "seems to leave us in the unhappy position of making imperative for infants treatments which many competent patients would decline for themselves—accepting for **all** infants what only **some** or, perhaps, **few** of the rest of us might accept for ourselves."[49]

Meilaender attempts a reconciliation of the two in offering the possibility that the kind and amount of treatment required for some spina bifida babies may well constitute burden **for the child** so severe that one might reasonably and morally forego further life-saving efforts even if the child is not yet irreversibly dying. Such a determination reflects more the burden-to-benefit proportionality of the ordinary/extraordinary means tradition than the physiologically-oriented "medical indications" policy of Ramsey. In short, Meilaender suggests, and this author tends to agree, that the child's best interest may be somewhat broader than Ramsey allows.

> Surely a parent, rather than focusing solely on physiological criteria, should be entitled to consider the emotional and psychological burdens (for the child) of treatment. If the child's "best interests" ought be narrowly construed because, as a child, it cannot determine one's best interests in any broader sense, "medically indicated" must be construed broadly enough to include emotional and psychological burdens.[50]

Meilaender concludes that while Ramsey's medical indications policy deals well with cases in which treatment is useless, it is less satisfactory in circumstances where treatment, although medically beneficial, is extraordinarily burdensome.

However, in the end Meilaender backtracks from this wider interpretation of an infant's best interest more to avoid a slippery slope to parental bias in practice than out of any conviction about the ethical illegitimacy of trans-biological burden factors.

> In a day when people seem to find it almost impossible to separate burdens for the child from burdens for the rest of us, Ramsey may be wise to construe a medical indications

policy rather narrowly. Perhaps his is, today, the only way to keep the child's best interests at the center of our concern. The possibility of abuse suggests that possibilities I discuss as appropriate might only serve as the "thin edge of the wedge" to prepare us for judgments of comparative worth of lives. If so, Ramsey's narrowly construed medical indications policy might still offer the best rule of practice for medicine to follow.[51]

Loyola University professor/pediatrician Eugene Diamond and U.S. Surgeon General C. Everett Koop are impassioned, compassionate, and somewhat polemical advocates of the right of handicapped infants to the fullest, most equitable treatment available.[52] Fearful of the "cult of perfection," in which a handicapped life is viewed as a fate worse than death, Koop and Diamond each cite numerous heroic examples of deformed and handicapped adults who value their own lives, "are glad that they were born," and "look forward to the future with hope and pleasant anticipation." Diamond champions the individualized, lowered expectation, person-oriented mindset of an institution for the handicapped like the Misericordia Home in Chicago in contradistinction to the "instant gratification" mentality of acute disease hospitals, in which "dramatic corrective surgery, resuscitative brinkmanship and rapid turnover of patients are their daily expectation."[53] Both Diamond and Koop raise the specter of Nazi Germany and the Third Reich's benign neglect and not so benign assault on "defective" newborns as a warning against the potential slippery slope inherent in refusing medically indicated therapeutic care based solely on the presence of some deformity or "defect." In three places Dr. Diamond paraphrases Ramsey's medical indications policy and praises it as "less susceptible to misuse in real world situations" than other alternatives.[54]

Responding somewhat precipitately to the perceived prejudicial decision made in the Bloomington Baby Doe Case, the Department of Health and Human Services, in May 1982, issued a 'medical indications'-based directive, which came to be known as the "Baby Doe Rule." Claiming authority under Section 504 of the Rehabilitation Act of 1973, the Department sent a notice to 6,800 federally subsidized hospitals declaring it unlawful "to withhold from a handicapped infant nutritional sustenance or medical or surgical treatment required to correct a life threatening condition," if the decision is based on the fact that the infant is handicapped, provided one's handicap does not render the procedure "medically contraindicated."[55]

Over the next ten months an Administration task force drafted fuller and stricter regulations, including a mandatory sign to be displayed in specific hospital locations and the establishment of a "hotline" to report suspected offenders. Opposed as alarmist and intrusive by the American Academy of Pediatrics and other plaintiffs, it was struck down by District Judge Gerhard Gesell, largely on procedural grounds, in April 1983. In July of that same year the DHHS attempted to implement a revised version, which set off another round of polarizing charges and counter-charges. Finally, Surgeon General C. Everett Koop, a respected conservative pediatrician, was allowed to attempt a compromise reworking of the DHHS regulations.[56]

Published in January 1984, this final version preserved the "medical indications" intent of the original notice, but with greater nuance, perhaps even some ambiguity of language. Accordingly, it was asserted that all "medically beneficial" treatment is obligatory and that "present or anticipated mental or physical impairment" (i.e., qualities of life) are invalid grist for nontreatment decision making. Paralleling both the content and much of the language of Ramsey's medical indications policy, the proposed regulations permitted withholding **only** those procedures judged clearly "futile," which "do no more than temporarily prolong the act of dying."[57] Two and a half years later, on June 9, 1986, the U.S. Supreme Court negated these DHHS Baby Doe Rules when it judged, in *Bowen v. American Hospital Association,* that Section 504 of the Rehabilitation Act of 1974 does not grant the federal government the authority to mandate nutritional or medically beneficial treatment for handicapped newborns.

This does not, however, negate Public Law 98-457 (October 9, 1984) nor its subsequent regulations for implementation, which in the interim had been hammered out as a compromise by both Houses of Congress in consultation with representatives of various advocacy groups.[58] This piece of legislation serves as a clarifying amendment to the Child Abuse and Neglect Act of 1974. It can be argued that this law, while refined and more carefully nuanced in its rules for implementation (April 15, 1985), still represents a legal victory for the medical indications position.

Before concluding this section surveying the components of a medical indications policy, it is necessary to discuss briefly a "thought experiment" begun by Ramsey in **The Patient as Person** and, despite nearly a decade of criticism, reaffirmed by him in **Ethics at the Edges of Life** with particular reference to severely handicapped infants.[59] Are there exceptions to the categorical imperative "never abandon care"? Irretrievably dying patients and incurable non-dying patients as a rule lay claim to our continued albeit non-curative "care" based on their inherent life and equality rights and our covenantal obligations to them. Is there ever moral justification for withholding even this basic hygienic, nutritional, and palliative care? Or, to go a step farther, is active infanticide ever exceptionally justified within a medical indications policy framework?

While Ramsey has consistently waged academic war against ethical relativism, his own ethical theory has not in all cases been rigidly deontological (i.e., prescriptive in an absolute sense). Borrowing the language and categories, if not all the content and nuance, from John Rawls' "Two Concepts of Rules," Ramsey developed two reasons for allowing rule "exceptions" to absolute norms.[60] The first validating reason is if the so-called "exception" is in fact a repeatable case and thus not a unique exception at all. Rather it constitutes a new species of action reflecting a new or unique rule, perhaps as a corollary to the former still exceptionless norm. The second example of an apparent exception would be cases in which one is in fact actually upholding the underlying principle or spiritual value behind the action rule while in deed breaking the letter of the law.

Ramsey posits two species of cases in which the categorical imperative "never abandon care" is superseded by the exempting new condition that "care" cannot be conveyed. Defining his understanding of care as a " 'role and relations' ethic" he raises the question whether there ever comes a time when care by a human agent no longer reaches the subject cared for. If such a time does come, "care" for the dying would become as useless as earlier further medical "cure" became futile. "A gift is not a gift unless received; care is not what we suppose unless received, even if minimally. If not at all, there is no obligation to continue to do the useless."[61] This reciprocal motif, which apparently hinges the duty to "care" on the recipient's ability to consciously accept such effort, appears to this author to contradict Ramsey's fundamental advocacy of covenantal fidelity, agapeic other-centered love, and loyalty to embodied human patients as persons on an egalitarian basis, regardless of their abilities or disabilities. However, Ramsey tends to speak of these "beyond care" patients as "dying" and asserts that if care, even in the most minimal form of human presence or touch, no longer reaches a patient, then there is no significant moral difference whether their deaths are accelerated by direct commission or merely not inhibited by omission of futile efforts.

Who fits this "beyond care" category? Ramsey suggests two generic types of cases—the permanently comatose and the intractably pained—and attempts to offer illustrations of each from the handicapped newborn domain. The first is **the patient in a deep, permanent coma,** beyond all sensory input, "utterly unreachable by any agent's care."[62] Ramsey continues to speak of these cases as "terminal patients," dying patients beyond care, although it is not altogether clear that "irreversible deep coma" and imminently "dying" are interchangeable terms, e.g., Karen Ann Quinlan. Responding to the critique that it may be impossible to judge if and when a patient is ever **totally** beyond the reach of a caring voice or touch, Ramsey bows in theory both to Helmut Thielicke's suggestion of a possible self-conscious passageway beyond human measure and to Hans Jonas' defense of the inviolability of an embodied human life.[63] And yet, in the realm of a "thought experiment," Ramsey need not populate the category with actual cases to still hold that **if** physicians can in fact determine the borderline between conscious living and permanently unconscious patients, the latter would be beyond care and the moral distinction between commission and omission would thereby be abrogated.

The lone neonatal candidate Ramsey mentions in relation to this category is the anencephalic infant, who earlier was labeled as "irretrievably dying" but still accessible to or at least deserving of human care while dying. Ramsey refines this with a two-pronged rationale for ceasing care and/or actively dispatching these anencephalic infants. First, adopting the definition of death as "the disintegration and ultimately the total absence of the natural functions of heart and lungs and brain," Ramsey defines the anencephalic infant as not merely dying at birth, but by definition not "alive." The absence of developed frontal lobes of the brain implies for Ramsey that systemic integration is absent even prior to delivery or "birth." The respect due them, he asserts, would be more like the respect to be given to the corpse of the deceased. He suggests that "one should be willing to 'kill' such brainless products of human generation if (contrary to the fact) they persisted in 'living' in that condition."[64] Much as one would act toward a decapitated chicken running around, one might mercifully stop or inhibit a "reflexively reacting corpse." Second, such "brainless" human infants are beyond care because lacking consciousness they cannot receive human input-love, tenderness, or the "warmth" of human presence. Impervious to human efforts, they are candidates either for nontreatment or for direct infanticide.

While Elizabeth MacMillan in no way condones active infanticide under any circumstances and while she does **not** define permanently comatose patients as already "dead," she does join Ramsey in suggesting that an "irreversibly unconscious" infant, whose cognitive upper brain is missing and/or permanently extinguished, may be classified as someone for whom further medical treatment is "medically infeasible" and thus optional.

> The infant at best will be able to breathe and perhaps to blink or swallow; it never will be able to see, feel, think, or otherwise relate to the outside world. Under such circumstances, few would argue that the available treatment actually benefits the child.[65]

It seems to me that MacMillan's interpretation reflects a humane yet subtle shift away from "the infant's physiological condition" toward a more holistic interpretation based on the infant's qualitative potential or lack thereof. Basing nontreatment decisions on one's incapacity for thought, feeling, and relatability seems to place upper brain function and quality-of-expected-life above maintenance of the lower brain stem and inherently valuable physiological life. MacMillan might have been more consistent to the medical indications or medical feasibility policy, and not altogether medically inaccurate, if she were to join Ramsey in defining such brain-defective, permanently unconscious patients as already embarked irretrievably upon the dying process, albeit over a longer, slower course. If an "irreversibly un-conscious" patient can be defined as already in the throes of death, then lack of thought, feeling, and relatability are only signs that one has already begun leave-taking from human, em-bodied living.

In addition to those patients who are permanently and deeply comatose, Ramsey suggests another species of patients for whom care is non-obligatory—**patients in intractable pain.** If it is medically impossible to keep excruciating physical pain at bay, then it is not incomprehensible to presume that a patient so tortured will be wholly absorbed in bodily agony, precluding any appreciable experience of human care or presence.[66] Asking whether there are any birth defects comparable to insurmount-able physiological pain, Ramsey posits, admittedly based on lim-ited knowledge, Lesch-Nyhan syndrome and epidermolysis bulloso (lethalis) as possible candidates. The genetic defect of Lesch-Nyhan syndrome, identified and described in a series of 1964 cases by Drs. Michael Lesch and William Nyhan, is passed on only to male infants. Victims suffer uncontrollable spasms and mental retardation, and are unable to walk or even to sit up unassisted. As these ultimately terminal and incurable infants reach the teething stage, they invariably begin gnawing on them-selves, mutilating lips, hands, shoulders, often biting off fingers or other appendages.

> Is this not a close approximation to the supposable case of insurmountable pain which in the terminal adult patient places him beyond human caring action and abolishes the moral significance of the distinction between always contin-uing to care and direct dispatch? When care cannot be con-veyed, it need not be extended.[67]

The relatively recent discovery of medication which promises to relieve the more horrible symptoms of this syndrome may bring it back within the domain of the obligation to care, while still leaving it an incurable and terminal genetic defect.

Ramsey believes the case of epidermolysis bulloso might serve as a better neonatal illustration of intractable pain warranting non-care or even direct "dispatch." According to Ramsey, any touching of the infant's genetically afflicted skin causes blisters, often large and prone to infection. Proper hospital care can heal the blisters, preparing the infant for a brief, sterile "touchless" life or, more likely, for a life plagued by recurring blisters caused by the very act of a caring touch. It is difficult to declare objectively if there is such a state as absolutely "intractable," "irremediable" and "insurmountable" pain. Reputable scholars line up on both sides of the issue.[68] So while this second class of patients who are beyond care may be a memberless group, Ramsey is not willing to baptize palliative drugs as necessarily alleviating all excruciating pain.

Lisa Sowle Cahill, a sympathetic commentator and critic of Ramsey's methodology, suggests that he might have been more consistent to the fundamental presuppositions of a medical indications policy, if he were to present these "exceptions" as deeper manifestations of the human dignity and covenantal loyalty principles underlying the norm "never abandon care." Cahill accepts Ramsey's presumption that such permanently comatose or insurmountably pained patients are generally already dying, not merely wretchedly living on, and states:

> We might say that the principle which grounds the rule "Do not kill" is "Respect Life." By gaining a deeper understanding of the sense of the principle itself, we find that some qualifications or "excuses" are built into its own authentic meaning. To make an exception to the prohibition against euthanasia, it seems that Ramsey would better argue that the present requirement of our covenant fidelity is to hasten the death of one already in the dying process. Respect for life could encompass direct euthanasia in some limited circum-

stances. This argument could claim consistency with the demands of both justice and love.[69]

Thereby a patient's receptivity is not the limiter or measure of parental, medical, and societal obligations to care. Still, such openness to euthanasia of the imminently dying would not justify directly causing the deaths of Lesch-Nyhan syndrome sufferers or of any other excruciatingly pained **non-dying** patients.

Ramsey acknowledges Cahill's methodological suggestions appreciatively, but is reluctant to shift his method of deriving euthanasia exceptions, lest labeling killing as "the caring thing to do" might grease the slippery slope to caring-motivated infanticide of incurable, pain-free, non-dying patients too.[70] Linking the possible use of euthanasia to a patient's condition and inability to benefit from the care rendered is more physiologically-based and parallels better the medical indications policy's criterion for foregoing useless curative treatment than linking killing to caring. For Ramsey, the latter borders too closely on quality-of-expected-life judgments by the agent about the voiceless patient's prospects for some subjective experience of "meaningful" life.

These controversial exceptions notwithstanding, a medical indications approach to nontreatment decisions, as advocated by Ramsey, MacMillan, et al., remains the strictest, most objective and medically focused of the non-vitalistic standards to be surveyed here. The American Academy of Pediatrics and a coalition of advocacy groups for handicapped persons' rights summarizes a "medical indications" policy succinctly in their "Principles of Treatment of Disabled Persons":

> When medical care is clearly beneficial, it should always be provided. . . . Consideration such as anticipated or actual limited potential of an individual and present or future lack

of available community resources are irrelevant and must not determine the decisions concerning medical care. The individual's medical condition should be the sole focus of the decision . . .

It is ethically and legally justified to withhold medical or surgical procedures which are clearly futile and will only prolong the act of dying. However, supportive care should be provided including sustenance as medically indicated and relief of pain and suffering . . .

In cases where it is uncertain whether medical treatment will be beneficial, a person's disability must not be the basis for a decision to withhold treatment. At all times during the process when decisions are being made about the benefit or futility of medical treatment, the person should be cared for in the medically most appropriate ways. When doubts exist at any time about whether to treat, a presumption always should be in favor of treatment.[71]

A "Medical Indications Policy"—A Critique

The critique section of this chapter will focus primarily on Paul Ramsey's presentation of a medical indications policy because his is the most thorough, ethically-oriented (as distinct from public policy), and theological elaboration of this normative standard. Ramsey and, by extension, all medical indications advocates are to be commended for their articulate and, at times, impassioned defense both of the inherent and equal dignity of every live-born member of the human species and of the moral claims that each human life thereby places on others—parents, health care personnel, and society—"to cure" and "to care." Judaeo-Christian belief and the U.S. Constitutional tradition both affirm that a living human being, however tragically handicapped, is and remains a **person**, a rights-bearing member of the moral community. This Ramsey forcefully argues against all encroachments by a Western society that he sees as increasingly prone to relativism, pure consequentialism, and utilitarianism. This inherent or innate approach to human worth and "person-hood" is in sharp contrast to some of the scholars to be surveyed in Chapter Four (Tooley, Singer), who evaluate human worth solely in terms of one's functional capabilities and/or social usefulness.

That said, however, medical indications proponents can rightly be faulted for so emphasizing one's inherent worth as a species member and so enshrining that value in **absolute** prescriptions for life-prolongation and proscriptions against cessation of life-sustaining therapies for "non-dying" patients, that the meaning of "life" and of "the patient's best interest" becomes truncated. In their zealous effort to forestall what they see as a purely functional bias against inherent rights or intrinsic values they have tended to confuse the absoluteness of the right to life and of its value with the kind of positive precept it calls forth. The best interest of the patient, rather than being rooted in one's physical embodiment, is in some sense reduced to it, or, at least in the cases of all salvageable patients, made subservient to it. Except in the cases of so-called "imminently dying" or incurable patients, for whom projected functional capabilities and social needs are allowed to influence the best course of humane care, Ramsey and his medical indications associates lean toward a domination of one's holistic best interest by one's embodiment and of one's total well-being by an anthropology too weighted toward the physical or biological.

The roots of this truncated view of the patient's best interests lie, for Ramsey, in his own Barthian-influenced, Protestant-based theology. Rather than viewing human persons as free-willed partners with God in the work of creation and unfolding redemption, Ramsey's sin-oriented, neo-orthodox mindset is more suspicious of human freedom. Accordingly, it is better to mandate prolongation of vital functions ("life" in its most basic physiological aspects), assuming that to be in the patient's best interest, than to trust redeemed (yet sinful) humanity to choose wisely. For Ramsey there is little continuity between God's creation of human life in the present and God's kingdom to come. The meantime, which Ramsey frequently refers to pejoratively in terms of Augustine's City of Man, seems discontinuous with one's future destiny, at least in terms of human cooperation or participation in bringing it about.[72] Therefore, absolute mandates to preserve "what is" seem preferable to risks for "what might be."

By contrast, the anthropology adopted by Thomas Aquinas and accepted in large measure by the Roman Catholic tradition espouses a more dynamic, multi-faceted concept of the human person and of his/her well-being. As with the medical indications approach, one's rights-bearing status as a person is grounded in one's very nature as a living member of the species. This serves to protect the life and inherent rights of those fellow persons who might otherwise be subjugated to some net social calculus. However, a patient's best interest or well-being is not restricted to the prolongation of life in its most basic or physiological aspects.

Human life as a whole or one's personhood is a dynamic reality, rooted in one's existence as an embodied being, but oriented toward "more." That "more" includes both penultimate human flourishing in terms of one's unique human potentialities for rationality and relationships as well as one's ultimate fulfillment in and with God hereafter. It is this "becoming" component that medical indications proponents tend to undervalue in their ardent defense of the intrinsic value of "being," life in its most basic physiological aspects. At best the two are sequentially related, the former being the pre-condition and valued basis for the latter. More often than not, prolongation of one's biological existence, "life" in the physiological sense, will be parallel to and constitutive of promoting one's wider best interest. However, the abiding obligation to respect the physiological aspects of one's life does not necessarily mean always prolonging vital signs if the other components of human flourishing are totally extinguished or will suffer because of it.

Just as a part or an organ within a living organism is ordered toward and subordinate to the smooth functioning and life of the organism as a whole, so also the various aspects of human well-being (the physical, psychological, social, and spiritual) are similarly ordered toward and ultimately subordinate to one's totality, the best interest of the person as an integrated whole. Bodily life, while a component of the earthly phase of one's human destiny, is not and ought not necessarily be the controlling element for a human person, whose interests and well-being are broader.

This Ramsey seems to acknowledge when he allows imminently dying patients or their caretakers to choose the "how" of living while dying that is best suited to one's psychological-social-spiritual well-being. So also, Ramsey's curious exceptions seem to indicate that the total cessation of one's embodied psychological and social abilities to experience is a sign that further life prolongation on the merely physiological level is no longer warranted. In each of these cases, Ramsey arguably permits trans-physiological or non-medical factors to determine the best interest of the patient. Only in the cases of so-called "non-dying" patients do medical indications proponents assume that prolonged biological life is necessarily desirable, in that patient's best interest, irrespective of the patient-centered burden caused or perpetuated. Only in these cases are sustained vital signs alone made synonymous with the best interests of the patient.

It might be argued in response that Ramsey in no way adopts a hierarchy of goods in which the physiological aspects of life are allowed to dominate one's human potential. Rather, Ramsey defends sustaining the physiological aspects of the lives of all patients not imminently dying because that is the essential pre-condition for and the most secure way of protecting those further dimensions of the patient's humanity. Thus, rather than reducing the personal or best interest to the physiological, Ramsey safeguards the former by a medical indications policy which mandates life-prolongation when it is medically feasible to do so.

That brings us back to the Ramsey quotation which opened this chapter: "Morally it is never right to turn against the good of human life." I agree wholeheartedly. The real question, however, is: What constitutes "the good of human life," particularly when it is historically enfleshed in a given patient? The scholars to be surveyed and critiqued in subsequent chapters will disagree with the medical indication presumption that prolonged physiological existence of all salvageable (i.e., not imminently dying) patients is necessarily a "respect life" decision in their best interest. **Burdens,** in terms of physical pain, mental anguish, a total loss of consciousness and relational potential, or even exorbitant resource costs for too little health gain, **may tragically outweigh** the generally assumed **benefit** of physiological life extension. While Ramsey and Sherlock assume this is a direct negation of the value of life, tantamount to throwing the gift of "life" back in the face of the Giver, it seems to the scholars to be presented in Chapters Two through Five that the best interest of the patient, especially given the technological fact that vital signs can be sustained almost indefinitely through the use of artificial life support equipment, ought to be broader. It ought to incorporate mental, relational and spiritual capacities (or lack thereof) in addition to the physical. If these are diminished severely or are even non-existent, then the value—**for the patient**—of medically feasible prolongation of his/her basic **bios** is proportionately less compelling, less obligatory, at times even contra-indicated.

With reference to "non-dying" patients medical indication proponents have absolutized both the positive prescription to sustain and prolong "life" in its physiological aspects as well as the negative proscription against the directly intended taking of innocent human life. Accordingly, they interpret all acts of non-prolongation in the cases of patients not imminently dying to be synonymous with directly intended euthanasia by omission. The medical ethics tradition would take issue with Ramsey, Sherlock, et al. on two points.

First of all, it has traditionally been recognized that one's duties to respect a fundamental right or value vary from **absolute negative precepts,** which categorically exclude certain choices as direct assaults on the right or value, to generally obligatory, **usually binding** (i.e., prima facie) **positive precepts,** which oblige one to foster the good insofar as it does not impinge on other obligations or disproportionately limit one's own rational and relational pursuits. In other words, the obligation to sustain or prolong **bios** is not as binding as the obligation not to kill or directly harm the physiological aspects of one's life, whether by acts of commission or directly intended omission.

Secondly, to choose to enhance the "how" or quality of one's life by refusing to impose burdens on a patient that would excessively inhibit his/her human flourishing, through a decision to forego means to prolong physiological "life," is not synonymous with morally intending or directly doing the deadly deed. One can choose **for** human well-being without thereby choosing **against** "life" in its fullness and without directly intending harm to "life" in its physiological aspects. Even within the medical indications schema, the choice to forego life-prolonging chemotherapy or life-sustaining respirators in the case of incurable, terminal patients reflects a choice for the patient's wider sense of well-being, not against "life" in any morally significant sense.

The more philosophical and legal advocates of a medical indications policy might well disavow any conscious affinity with all this talk of opposing Christian interpretations of one's spiritual or ultimate best interest. However, the common medical indications policy fear of the abuse of handicapped persons in the here and now bespeaks a secular parallel to the religious language above. In an effort to forestall any possible abuse, medical indications advocates have tried to jettison the determination of non-medical (i.e., non-physiological) burden altogether, except in very restricted, potentially inconsistent instances. What is left is a physiologically-restricted standard, which defends saving and prolonging vital signs as mandatory for all non-dying, treatable patients. To mandate salvaging and prolonging every human life that is not imminently dying or untreatable may be to defend the intrinsic value of "life" in its physiological aspects at the expense of a patient's total well-being, "Life" in a fuller sense. This criticism will hopefully become more apparent as we deal with specific case applications.

Medical indications proponents are to be commended for allowing the parents of so-called irreversibly, imminently dying infants to withhold or withdraw further futile therapies, shifting over to humane care and psychological support. They are to be commended for accepting the body's own "rhythm of life" by not mandating artificially maintained vital signs when the patient's brain has no potential for regaining integrated control over such functions. Likewise, medical indications proponents are to be commended for seeing that useless therapies on incurable conditions serve only to waste resources or perhaps to exacerbate the medical problem and are thus optional, even "medically contra-indicated." All the scholars to be surveyed in the chapters to come will concur with the decision to forego treatment in these cases. If a proposed treatment offers no bodily benefit in terms of cure or if a life-sustaining device is no longer a component within a wider program of therapeutic cure, but merely forestalls the imminently inevitable, then such procedures are optionally unwarranted. In some cases that option may yield to contra-indication, particularly if the patient is suffering or if someone else with a prognosis for medical benefit is being deprived of the use of the equipment or funds.

By way of illustration, all medical indications proponents

agree that the infant born with anencephaly is imminently dying, with death likely to occur in a matter of hours, days, or, at most, weeks. Further futile therapies or mere life-sustainers are "medically contra-indicated." On the other hand, Tay Sachs or Lesch-Nyhan infants, who are terminal or "dying" in the long term sense (possibly five years), are not judged to be "imminently" so. Therefore, interim therapies on the symptoms of their terminal condition and on other semi-related life-threatening problems would be "medically indicated." So far, so good.

But what about Trisomy 13 or 18 infants? Born with massive, incurable brain deficiencies, these children fall on the spectrum between anencephalic infants with a life expectancy of hours or days and infants with Tay Sachs disease or Lesch-Nyhan syndrome. Six months to a year of life is often possible for these relatively non-conscious babies, especially if respiration and feeding are assisted as needed and infections and pneumonia are kept at bay. Elizabeth MacMillan readily included these infants in the category of those irreversibly and imminently dying.[73] Ramsey's impassioned assertion that "six months of babyhood" ought not be judged of less ultimate value than "sixty years of manhood or womanhood" seems to indicate that for him death might not be "imminent" enough in these cases to allow for withholding antibiotics, minor surgeries, and respiratory therapies.[74]

In an attempt to forestall quality of life judgments about the relative or subjective worth of prolonging a given infant's life, medical indications proponents attempt to articulate objective physiological categories, as if membership in one or another automatically demands a different species of care. Ramsey puts great stock in the supposed medical distinction between "dying" and "non-dying" for determining when neonatal treatment may be contraindicated. University of Virginia ethicist James Childress challenges this when he asserts that "it is not clear that Ramsey's distinction between dying and non-dying can carry as much freight as he loads on it."[75] I would expand this criticism of the "dying" vis-à-vis "non-dying" distinction to include the similarly fluid distinctions between someone "imminently dying" and someone facing "a longer term, incurable, terminal illness," between merely "prolonging dying" and "prolonging life," and between being "beyond care" and being "minimally within the reach of care."[76]

Admitting for the sake of prudential medical decision making that physicians attempt to make such judgments, Ramsey seems willing to hinge qualitatively different species of treatment on these imprecise lines of demarcation.[77] The problem is that Trisomy 13 and 18 babies, for example, fall between the cracks unless someone defines "imminent" more precisely in terms of time length—what constitutes imminent as distinct from distant dying? As Stanley Hauerwas phrases it, "how long do you have to live to be a 'liver' rather than a 'dier'?"[78] So also, when in the four to five year life span of a Lesch-Nyhan syndrome baby or one with Tay Sachs disease may one declare such an irreversibly incurable and terminal child to be "imminently" in the throes of death? Prior to such a sign-off point one would arguably be obliged to aggressively treat all infections, flus, urinary or bowel disorders, heart defects, respiratory ailments, and orthopedic complications to enhance the physiological quality of the child's terminal existence. Only at the point when s/he is declared "imminently" dying may one cease such efforts, presumably in the patient's wider best interest, to forestall death from the major anomaly or even from those semi-unrelated medical problems that heretofore were aggressively treated. It seems that the spectrum from irreversibly imminently dying through irreversibly dying through terminal through incurable through merely handicapped is far too fluid and imprecise to make the kind of treatment that is ethically mandatory hinge on one's classification in one or another of these categories.

In a sense this is a species of the "Technical Criteria Fallacy" outlined by Robert Veatch. Referring specifically to the

Apgar Score used to determine whether resuscitation of a minutes-old infant will be prognostically beneficial and to Lorber's six physiological criteria for determining on day one of life whether a myelomeningocele newborn will benefit from treatment, Veatch defines this fallacy:

> It is not the precise content of the list which is important. Rather it is the concept that **any** list of objectively measurable criteria can be translated directly into decisions about selection for treatment and nontreatment. Presumably the lists being proposed are meant to be reasonably accurate measures of prognoses. Yet the presumption that treatment or nontreatment rests solely on prognosis is surely contestable. The decision must also include evaluation of the meaning of existence with varying impairments.[79]

Veatch goes on to suggest that those who advocate treatment for all or practically all newborns might be committing a species of the technical criteria fallacy. The technical ability to accumulate data and tally scores ought not be deemed synonymous with the ethical imperative, both because such raw data requires fallible, value-laden interpretation and because a patient's holistic best interest ought to incorporate **more** than biological prognosis.

Two flaws are contained in a medical indications standard which bases nontreatment decisions so heavily on medical diagnosis/prognosis and on the inclusion of an infant in one or another biological category of patients. First, as noted above, such physiologically-based categories are fluid, imprecise, and based in many instances on "guesstimates," the art of prudential medical discernment or prognoses, not exact science. Basing life-saving treatment or its rejection solely on one's membership in such imprecise categories lends itself to the abuse of borderline patients. Second, and even more fundamental, is the real or more universalizable reason for ceasing further interim therapies in the cases of imminently dying or incurable patients actually based so singly on their physiological condition? Is it not rather a more value-laden decision that, given the relative **though not absolute** futility of further curative efforts or of merely life-sustaining devices, life prolongation in a biological sense may not be worth it to the patient in terms of pain, suffering, and cost—"burden" in the more holistic sense?

For the so-called irreversibly, imminently dying patient and for the patient with a major untreatable handicap, the focus of future treatment and care seems to have transcended purely physiological concerns. Given the fact that almost every infant could be kept biologically "alive" indefinitely through the use of respirators and heart pumps, the non-vitalistic willingness of medical indications proponents to "pull the plug" in certain cases indicates some value or respect for the well-being of the human patient that overrides mere **bios** prolongation. More importantly, the decision to forego potentially beneficial interim therapies, such as chemotherapy, radiation, insulin, and antibiotics, in the cases of some patients nearer death implies that the quality of life while dying outweighs its mere prolongation quantitatively-speaking.

> Strictly speaking, there is medical benefit to treatment which, though it cannot cure, can extend life even briefly. To choose, in one's way of dying, to refuse such treatment is to do so not because it lacks benefit, but because it lacks **sufficient** benefit. This matter of **sufficient** benefit opens the door once again to indications which are not strictly medical.[80]

"Medically feasible" and "morally indicated" ought not be synonymous. The former refers to technological capability and biological sustainability, while the latter is a more inclusive concept, situating the merit or demerit of this feasibility within the context of the patient's holistic well-being. Just as a patient irretrievably close to death may opt for hospice-like care and a shorter lifespan instead of a minimal yet medically feasible extension of the physiological aspects of life, so also I suggest that such is and ought to be the case with every patient, whether dying, terminal, incurable, or merely horribly handicapped.

Related to this is the potential inconsistency between the non-medical factors that Ramsey seems willing to allow competent patients to bring to bear in treatment decisions and his categorical rejection of such factors where non-competent newborns are concerned. It appears that, for Ramsey, competent patients in some sense retain their right to incorporate personal psychological, social, and religious factors into medical decisions with the possibility that some combination might yield a non-treatment decision, overriding what is medically indicated in a strictly physiological sense.[81] However, with reference to handicapped newborns Ramsey judges such burden-over-benefit judgments as prejudicial and **a priori** not in the patient's best interest. Meilaender, Cahill, McCormick, and Arras all note Ramsey's inconsistency here.[82] As Jesuit John Connery phrases it, "Is it reasonable to make incompetent people bear burdens that competent people do not have to bear?"[83] It is not my purpose here to highlight Ramsey's inconsistencies nor to settle the haziness of his rhetoric regarding competent patients, non-medical burdens, and an agent's freedom. Rather, it is sufficient to say that his unwillingness to **categorically** reject all burden components, particularly for competent patients, bespeaks some recognition that medical feasibility is not synonymous with what is morally indicated. Whether one shies away from the language of quality of life or not, some trans-biological or qualitative components do impact on decisions to forego treatment despite projected degrees of medical benefit and feasibility.

Hidden within a medical indications standard, however subtly or unintentionally, are the seeds or perhaps the echoes of a broader, more holistic view of the patient's best interest. The very rejection of absolute vitalism indicates that the value, meaning, or ultimate worth of human life for medical indications proponents transcends the feasibility of merely sustaining respiration and circulation. Medical indications proponents go on to allow such trans-biological or holistic factors to override minimally beneficial means in certain cases. Future chapters will take up this question further: In addition to medical (i.e., physiological) feasibility, what other patient-centered or even non-patient factors ought to be considered before deciding that a certain procedure is or is not morally indicated? Appreciating and even concurring with the "fears" concerning potential bias against the handicapped, I wonder if the medical indications policy solution might not also be excessive and "fearsome" in the opposite direction. The **forced** life-saving or life-prolonging treatment of some few borderline salvageable infants, whose lives are generally perceived as wretched and extraordinarily burdened, may well offset the justice focus of this medical indications policy with another species of injustice.

On at least two occasions Ramsey has taken up the case of Karen Ann Quinlan, a young woman whose seemingly permanent comatose state (from 1975 until her death in 1985) made her in many ways a parallel non-competent patient to some severely brain-damaged newborns.[84] Prior to her 1976 weaning from a respirator, Ramsey presumed, as did the official medical prognosis, that Ms. Quinlan was irreversibly, imminently dying. Out of respect for the patient's best interest Ramsey suggested that tube or I.V. feeding be ceased at the same time that she was taken off the respirator, since both respirator and artificially administered nourishment were merely prolonging the irreversible dying process. To everyone's surprise, Ms. Quinlan continued to breathe on her own once the respirator was removed. Her parents declined to follow Ramsey's suggestion concerning the withdrawal of artificially assisted nourishment. As the years passed one might argue that Karen Ann had become a candidate for Ramsey's "beyond care" category, but he could no longer classify her, a nine year respirator alumna, as "imminently dying." Aware of the compassion Ramsey has shown for Quinlan and her family, ethicist Richard McCormick asked whether Ramsey would now demand that a "non-dying" Karen be put back on a respirator if the need arose to tide her over a temporary pneumonia crisis.[85] A strict medical indications policy would necessarily conclude that if she is only incurable and/or terminal, but not imminently dying, what can be done ought to be done to save and prolong her biological life.

The criticism exemplified here is this. The value to the patient of treatment to correct a life-threatening condition need not and ought not be made in a biological vacuum, as if that medical problem is distinct from the composite picture of the patient's physiological-mental condition. In the case of a Trisomy 21 infant with duodenal atresia, the criticism of the decision to withhold treatment is not so much the assertion that one ought to categorically prescind from incorporating the child's mental condition into the ethical equation, but rather that in this case Down's Syndrome is not a brain deficiency of significant enough magnitude to inhibit the technological success or holistic value **for the patient** of the proposed surgery. However, if one's mental handicap is of such severity that the patient is terminal, even if not imminently so, does that not color the decision concerning interim therapies on affected organ systems, the origin of which usually cannot be separated from the child's fundamental developmental "defect"? Or in the case of infants whose deaths from underlying long-term terminal anomalies will be excruciating or torturous, as is the case with Lesch-Nyhan syndrome or epidermolysis bulloso, is it necessary to approach related medical problems (infections, pneumonia, etc.) as if the underlying condition and the projected painful dying process do not exist? Conscious of the safeguard needed against flippant prejudice against the mildly or manageably retarded based solely on their "substandard" mental capacities, the solution ought not be to compartmentalize one's anomalies and diseases as if they do not impact as a totality both on that patient's physiological health and on his/her total well-being.

We have now come full circle back to Baby Boy Houle. It seems that Judge Roberts wrongly dissected the infant into isolated diseases and treatments. The medical feasibility of removing the boy's tracheal esophageal fistula was set apart from his multiple other birth defects. It can rightly be debated whether being cycloptic, blind, half-deaf, facially disfigured, digitally malformed, partially paralyzed, and brain-damaged actually constitutes extraordinary burden or a quality of life beyond reasonable benefit. However, to prescind from the reality of this list of physiological factors as part of this infant's total diagnosis and prognosis, let alone from some projection of burden to come, is potentially an equally gross species of injustice.

Finally, some brief comment should be made concerning Ramsey's "curious exceptions." While sympathetic to Ramsey's inclination to exempt permanently non-conscious or intractably pained patients from the obligation to sustain or prolong such "unresponsive," even tortured lives, one must question if he is being consistent to his own fundamental principles. If every "individual human life is absolutely unique, inviolable, irreplaceable, non-interchangeable, not substitutable and not meldable with other lives" and if one's functional ability or relational potential ought to have no bearing on what is medically feasible and thereby indicated for the non-dying patient, how can he declare some inherently worthwhile, presumably personal lives to be "beyond care," with no abiding claim on parents or society to respect their intrinsically valuable personhood or "life"?[86]

If he were to adopt Lisa Cahill's suggestion that nontreatment (or even active infanticide) is "the caring thing to do," that is, in the tragically handicapped newborn's best interest, then Ramsey might claim to be consistent with his inherent/equal worth premises, though such a shift would do further damage to his supposedly physiologically-oriented medical indications policy.[87] As it is, Ramsey seems to purchase these two curious exceptions at too great a price—the negation of his own fundamental assertion that human life, irrespective of consciousness, relationality, or level of burden is personal, inherently of value, absolutely inviolable. If "beyond care" is synonymous with the assertion that a patient's "life" so designated no longer has rightful claims on our care, then, in some sense, Ramsey has depersonalized these most tragic patients. They lose their fundamental equality with other living human beings and, by definition, are either non-persons or, at least, lesser persons.

In light of Ramsey's previous defense of the intrinsic worth of every live-born member of the human species, it would be far better to declare such tragically handicapped patients to be persons, inherently valuable subjects deserving our continued care, and then to make decisions in their total best interest, seen in psychological, social, and spiritual as well as physiological terms. Whether active euthanasia would ever be deemed in their best interest (e.g., intractably pained infant) is a moral question for another study, but at least it would then be raised in the context of the patient as person, even if beyond the conscious reach of care.

Ramsey's curious exceptions are some of the very cases which lead the scholars to be surveyed in succeeding chapters to judge a medical indications standard inadequate. Permanently unconscious patients, while probably terminal in some long-range sense, are not imminently dying and therefore would not generally fit within the medical indications parameters for non-treatment of life-threatening problems that arise. So also, an intractably pained patient, perhaps exemplified by an infant with epidermolysis bulloso, is tragically plagued, but hardly imminently dying. Pain medication unto suppression of respiration might be condoned under the direct/indirect distinction, but it is doubtful that a "pure" medical indications standard could accept the abandonment of life-sustenance for this non-dying patient. After all, would they not say that "life" in a biological sense, even if tragically pained, is of incalculable value?

The scholars to be surveyed in the following chapters will answer this question with varying degrees of a nuanced "no." For all of them Ramsey's curious exceptions are indicative of the hard cases in which other trans-physiological values must be brought to bear. Ramsey exempted these cases from his medical indications standard and in the process borders on contradicting and undermining his own system. Would it not be preferable to broaden the method and widen the criteria to deal more consistently with the permanently non-conscious, the intractably pained, and others whose wider well-being may rightly outweigh the value—for the patient—of "mere" bios-prolongation?

In summary, Ramsey, MacMillan, Sherlock, Dyck, Diamond, and Koop are to be commended for their eloquent articulation of fears about creeping subjective autonomy, utilitarianism, and a perfectionist bias against the handicapped in our society. More accolades are due proponents of a medical indications policy for their defense of inherent rights and corresponding duties against pure consequentialism or social utilitarianism. These qualified compliments notwithstanding, ultimately a medical indications policy is too restrictive and thus inadequate to the task of determining when to withhold or withdraw treatment from severely handicapped newborns. Weak on the psychological, social, and spiritual aspects of a fuller Christian/human concept of the patient's well-being, medical indications advocates adopt a policy in which a more restrictive and somewhat physicalistic notion tends to dominate one's best interests, particularly in the case of "non-dying" patients. As Lisa Sowle Cahill concisely states in her review of **Ethics at the Edges of Life**:

> Ramsey's proposal of a physical standard of benefit and
> therefore of "medically indicated" treatment may purchase
> objectivity at the price of a more refined ethical sensitivity to
> the [fuller] needs of the most vulnerable claimers of care.[88]

Ironically, these "most vulnerable claimers of care" are the very
patients that a medical indications standard is designed to protect. A newborn's best interest, which should be a (the?) primary
focus of what is ethically indicated, is and rightly should be wider
than medical feasibility. What is physiologically beneficial and,
in that sense, "medically indicated" constitutes only phase one
of a multi-layered ethical process, regardless of a patient's competence or non-competence. Reduction of ethics to physiology
is clearer, seemingly safer, and certainly less prone to quality of
life abuses, but ultimately inadequate to the "human" ethical
task.

NOTES

[1]State of Maine, Superior Court, Cumberland County,
"Maine Medical Center vs. Houle, Opinion and Order," Superior Court Civil Action Docket #74-145 (February 14, 1974),
pp. 2–3; Ronald M. Soskin and S. John Vitello, "Defective Newborns: A Right to Treatment or a Right to Die?" **Amicus** 4 (May/
June 1979), p. 124; Leonard J. Weber, **Who Shall Live?** (New
York: Paulist Press, 1976), p. 13. According to Weber the child
was given the name "David Patrick," though all other sources
refer to him generically as "Baby Boy Houle."

[2]Maine, Superior Court, "Maine Medical Center vs.
Houle," p. 4.

[3]Paul Ramsey, **Ethics at the Edges of Life: Medical and
Legal Intersections** (New Haven: Yale University Press, 1978),

pp. 154–155, 178, 188; Elizabeth S. MacMillan, "Birth-Defective Infants: A Standard for Nontreatment Decisions," **Stanford Law Review** 30 (February 1978), p. 623.

[4]Paul Ramsey, "The Sanctity of Life—In the First of It," **The Dublin Review** 511 (Spring 1967), pp. 3–23; Ramsey, "On (Only) Caring for the Dying," **The Patient as Person: Explorations in Medical Ethics** (New Haven: Yale University Press, 1970), pp. 113–164. Also of help in devising a Medical Indications policy are the Preface and opening pages of Chapter One, pp. xi–xxii, 1–11; Ramsey, "Prolonged Dying: Not Medically Indicated," **Hastings Center Report** 6 (February 1976), pp. 14–17; Ramsey, "Euthanasia and Dying Well Enough," **Linacre Quarterly** 44 (February 1977), pp. 37–46; Ramsey, **Ethics at the Edges of Life**, pp. xi–xvii, 143–268; Ramsey, "Introduction," in **Infanticide and the Handicapped Newborn,** eds. Horan and Delahoyde, pp. vii–xvi; Elizabeth S. MacMillan, "Birth-Defective Infants: A Standard for Nontreatment Decisions," **Stanford Law Review** 30 (February 1978), pp. 599–633.

[5]Coalition of American Academy of Pediatricians, et al., "Principles of Treatment of Disabled Infants," **Pediatrics** 73 (4 April 1984), pp. 559–560; Dennis J. Horan, "Euthanasia, Medical Treatment and the Mongoloid Child: Death as a Treatment of Choice?" **Baylor Law Review** 27 (Winter 1975), pp. 76–85; Dennis J. Horan and David Mall, eds., **Death, Dying, and Euthanasia** (Washington, D.C.: University Publications of America, 1977); K. Hull, **The Rights of Physically Handicapped People: An American Civil Liberties Union Handbook** 22 (1979).

[6]Betty Lou Dotson, "Notice to Health Care Providers," **Federal Register** 47 (June 16, 1982): 26027. See note 8 of previous chapter for a fuller note on the "Baby Doe Rule."

[7]Ramsey, **Ethics at the Edges of Life**, p. xiv; Reflects the

same sentiments as Karl Barth, "Respect for Life" and "The Protection of Life" in **Church Dogmatics,** 4 vols. (Edinsburgh: T & T Clark, 1961), 3/4, pp. 324–470.

[8]Daniel J. Callahan, "The Sanctity of Life," in **Updating Life and Death,** ed. Donald R. Cutler (Boston: Beacon Press, 1969), pp. 223–250.

[9]"United Nations' Declaration of Human Rights—Preamble," in **The International Bill of Human Rights** (Glen Ellen, Ill.: Entwhistle Books, 1981), p. 3.

[10]Ramsey, **The Patient as Person,** p. xiii; a similar view is expressed in Ramsey, "The Sanctity of Life," p. 10.

[11]Ramsey, **Ethics at the Edges of Life,** pp. 146–147.

[12]Richard Sherlock, "Selective Non-Treatment of Defective Newborns: A Critique," **Ethics in Science and Medicine** 7 (1980), p. 112; Richard Sherlock, **Preserving Life: Public Policy and the Life Not Worth Living** (Chicago: Loyola University Press, 1987), p. 82.

[13]Ramsey, "The Sanctity of Life," p. 10; MacMillan, "Birth-Defective Infants," p. 619. Triage situations in the time of war or (inter)national crisis serve as necessary exceptions to this generally exceptionless norm.

[14]American Academy of Pediatricians, et al., "Principles of Treatment of Disabled Infants," p. 559: "Discrimination of any type against any individual with a disability/disabilities, regardless of the nature or severity of the disability, is morally and legally indefensible. Throughout their lives, all disabled individuals have the same rights as other citizens, including access to such major social activities as health care, education, and employment."

[15]Soskin and Vitello, "Defective Newborns," p. 122.

[16]Ramsey, **Ethics at the Edges of Life,** p. 205. Here the term "universal" tends to mean within one's cultural milieu, though global equity should be a long-range justice goal.

[17]Paul Ramsey, **Fabricated Man** (New Haven: Yale University Press, 1970), p. 119; Ramsey, **The Patient as Person,** pp. xii, 2, 5–11, 160; Ramsey, "Some Rejoinders," **Journal of Religious Ethics** 4 (Fall 1976), p. 191; Ramsey, **Ethics at the Edges of Life,** pp. xiii–xiv; It might be appropriate to note here that a number of Ramsey's commentators and critics point to a shift in his writing across the last two decades from an ethic based on Agapeic duty, which is wholly one-sided, to one built on Covenant fidelity, which seems to take into account mutuality and duty limits. See Paul F. Camenisch, "Paul Ramsey's Task: Some Methodological Clarifications and Questions," in **Love and Society,** eds. James Johnson and David Smith (Missoula, Mont.: Scholars Press, 1974), pp. 67–89; Charles E. Harris, Jr., "Love as the Basic Moral Principle in Paul Ramsey's Ethics," **Journal of Religious Ethics** 4 (Fall 1978), pp. 239–258; Lisa Sowle Cahill, "Paul Ramsey: Covenant Fidelity in Medical Ethics," **Journal of Religion** 55 (October 1975), pp. 470–476; Lisa Sowle Cahill, "Within Shouting Distance: Paul Ramsey and Richard McCormick on Method," **Journal of Medicine and Philosophy** 4 (1979), pp. 398–417; Charles E. Curran, **Politics, Medicine, and Christian Ethics: A Dialogue with Paul Ramsey** (Philadelphia: Fortress Press, 1973), esp. pp. 147–163; Joseph L. Allen, "Paul Ramsey and His Respondents Since the Patient as Person," **Religious Studies Review** 5 (1979), pp. 89–95.

[18]MacMillan, "Birth-Defective Infants," p. 619.

[19]Ramsey, **The Patient as Person,** p. 2.

[20] Paul Ramsey, **Basic Christian Ethics** (New York: Charles Scribners Sons, 1950), Dedication + pp. xi, 13, 107,

115–116, 124, 130; Ramsey, **Deeds and Rules in Christian Ethics** (New York: Charles Scribners Sons, 1967), pp. 108–109; Ramsey, **Fabricated Man,** pp. 29–31; Ramsey, **The Patient as Person,** pp. xii–xiii, 2, 25, 58, 256; Paul Ramsey, **The Ethics of Fetal Research,** pp. xiii, xv–xvi, 218.

[21]Charles E. Curran, "Utilitarianism and Contemporary Moral Theology: Situating the Debates," in **Readings in Moral Theology No. 1: Moral Norms and Catholic Tradition,** eds. Charles E. Curran and Richard A. McCormick, S.J. (New York: Paulist Press, 1979), pp. 341–362. This article originally appeared under the same title in **Louvain Studies** 6 (1977), pp. 239–255 and was reprinted as Chapter 5 in Charles E. Curran, **Themes in Fundamental Moral Theology** (Notre Dame: University of Notre Dame Press, 1977), pp. 121–144; Richard A. McCormick, "Reflections on the Literature," in **Readings in Moral Theology No. 1: Moral Norms and Catholic Tradition,** pp. 318–319. This article is a compilation from McCormick's "Notes on Moral Theology"—1972, 1975, 1977, 1978—from **Theological Studies;** William E. May, "Ethics and Human Identity: The Challenge of the New Biology," **Horizons** 3 (1976), p. 29.

[22]Ramsey, **Ethics at the Edges of Life,** pp. 154ff.

[23]Ibid., p. 158.

[24]Ibid., pp. 160–171; Robert M. Veatch, **Death, Dying, and the Biological Revolution: Our Last Quest for Responsibility** (New Haven: Yale University Press, 1976), pp. 77–163, esp. p. 110; Veatch, "Guardian Refusal of Life-Saving Medical Procedures: The Standard of Reasonableness," unpublished paper cited by Ramsey, p. 161.

[25]Veatch, **Death, Dying, and the Biological Revolution,** pp. 117–118.

[26]Ramsey, **Ethics at the Edges of Life,** pp. 158–159; Ramsey, "Prolonged Dying: Not Medically Indicated," p. 15.

[27]Ramsey, **Ethics at the Edges of Life,** pp. 171–181; MacMillan, "Birth-Defective Infants," pp. 620–623; Sherlock, "Selective Non-Treatment of Newborns," pp. 139–142; Sherlock, "Selective Non-Treatment of Defective Newborns: A Critique," pp. 111–117; Sherlock, "Public Policy and the Life Not Worth Living," pp. 121–132; Sherlock, **Preserving Life,** pp. 12–13, 106; Soskin and Vitello, "Defective Newborns," pp. 121–123; Arthur Dyck, "Ethical Reflections on Infanticide," in **Infanticide and the Handicapped Newborn,** esp. pp. 107–108, 114–120.

[28]Sherlock, "Selective Non-Treatment of Defective Newborns," p. 113.

[29]MacMillan, "Birth-Defective Infants," pp. 619, 622–623; Soskin and Vitello, "Defective Newborns," pp. 120–122; Sherlock, "Selective Non-Treatment of Defective Newborns," p. 116.

[30]Ramsey, **Ethics at the Edges of Life,** pp. 171–181.

[31]Ibid., p. 159. In an article entitled "Prolonged Dying: Not Medically Indicated" (1976), a precursor to pages 153–160 of **Ethics at the Edges of Life,** Ramsey "suggested that the morally significant meaning of ordinary and extraordinary medical means can be reduced almost without remainder to two components"—a comparison of treatments to determine if they are "medically indicated" and a patient's right to refuse treatment (p. 15). Yet in his 1978 revised presentation of this premise, Ramsey is careful to nuance the latter, restricting the right to refuse lest autonomous license ensue. A medical indications policy is left once the right to refuse is restricted to a right to refuse only those treatments not medically indicated anyway.

[32]Ibid., pp. 154–155.

[33]Ramsey, **The Patient as Person**, pp. 125, 132; Ramsey, **Ethics at the Edges of Life**, pp. 156, 178, 195.

[34]Ramsey, **Ethics at the Edges of Life**, p. 178.

[35]Ibid., p. 187.

[36]MacMillan, "Birth-Defective Infants," pp. 610–618, 628–629; Ramsey is less clear on the locus of decision-making, relying more heavily on the physician's determination of "dying" or of potential "medical benefit," but he does speak of parental consent in the child's behalf: Ramsey, **The Patient as Person**, pp. 26, 143; Ramsey, **Ethics at the Edges of Life**, p. 202.

[37]Interview with Dr. Anne Fletcher, Director of Neonatal ICU, Children's Hospital National Medical Center, Washington, D.C., 16 January 1984.

[38]Ramsey, **Ethics at the Edges of Life**, pp. 194, 192.

[39]Ibid., p. 165.

[40]Ibid., p. 206; and Ramsey, "Two-Step Fantastic: The Continuing Case of Brother Fox," **Theological Studies** 42 (March 1981), p. 133.

[41]Ramsey, **Ethics at the Edges of Life**, pp. 181–188; R. B. Zachary, "Ethical and Social Aspects of Treatment of Spina Bifida," **Lancet** 2 (1968), pp. 274–276; Zachary, "The Challenge of Spina Bifida," Editorial, **Journal of the All India Institute of Medical Science**, New Delhi (April 1976); Zachary, "Paediatric Surgery and Legislation: Congenital Aonomalies—A Rational Basis for Treatment," Paper delivered at European Congress of Catholic Doctors, May, 24, 1976; Zachary, "The Neonatal Surgeon," The Forshall Lecture, 23rd International Congress of Pediatric Surgeons, July 9, 1976 in **British Medical Journal** 280

(October 9, 1976), pp. 866–869; Zachary, "Life with Spina Bifida," **British Medical Journal** 281 (December 9, 1977), pp. 1460–1462; Zachary, "To Save or Let Die," **Tablet** 232 (February 1978), pp. 174–175; Zachary, "Give Every Baby a Chance," in "Spina Bifida: To Treat or Not To Treat?" **Nursing Mirror** 147 (September 14, 1978), pp. 13–19; Zachary and Sydney Brandon, "Operation on Infant with Down's Syndrome," **Lancet** 2 (September 12, 1981), p. 586.

[42]Zachary, "Life with Spina Bifida," p. 1460; Zachary, "Give Every Baby a Chance," p. 17; Chester Swinyard, ed., **Decision-making and the Defective Newborn: Proceedings of a Conference on Spina Bifida and Ethics** (Springfield, Ill.: Charles C. Thomas, 1978).

[43]Ramsey, **Ethics at the Edges of Life,** pp. 193–194; John Lorber, "Results of Treatment of Myelomeningocele: An Analysis of 524 Unselected Cases, with Special Reference to Possible Selection for Treatment," **Developmental Medicine and Child Neurology** 13 (1971), pp. 279–303; Lorber, "Spina Bifida Cystica: Results of Treatment of 270 Consecutive Cases with Criteria for Selection for the Future," **Archives of Disease in Childhood** 47 (1972), pp. 854–873; Lorber, "Early Results of Selective Treatment of Spina Bifida Cystica," **British Medical Journal** 277 (1973), pp. 201–204; Lorber, "Selective Treatment of Myelomeningocele: To Treat or Not To Treat," **Pediatrics** 53 (1974), pp. 307–308; Lorber, "Ethical Problems in the Management of Myelomeningocele and Hydrocephalus," **Journal of the Royal College of Physicians** 10 (October 1975), pp. 47–52; also in **Nursing Times** 72 (February 26, 1976), pp. 5–8 and (March 25, 1976), pp. 9–11; Lorber, "Spina Bifida: To Treat or Not To Treat?" **Nursing Mirror** 47 (September 14, 1978), pp. 13–19.

[44]Zachary, "Life with Spina Bifida," p. 1461; Zachary, "Give

Every Baby a Chance," pp. 17–18; Zachary, "To Save or Let Die," p. 174.

[45]Zachary, "To Save or Let Die," p. 175; Ramsey, **Ethics at the Edges of Life,** pp. 185–186.

[46]Arthur Dyck, "Ethical Reflections on Infanticide," in **Infanticide and the Handicapped Newborn,** eds. Horan and Delahoyde, p. 108; Dyck, **On Human Care: An Introduction to Ethics** (Nashville: Abingdon Press, 1977), p. 85; also by Dyck on the topic: Dyck, "An Alternative to the Ethics of Euthanasia," in **To Live and To Die,** ed. Robert H. Williams (New York: Springer-Verlag, 1973), pp. 98–112; Dyck, "The Good Samaritan Ideal and Beneficent Euthanasia: Conflicting Views of Mercy," **Linacre Quarterly** 42 (August 1975), pp. 176–188; Dyck, "Beneficent Euthanasia and Benemortasia: Alternative Views of Mercy," in **Beneficent Euthanasia,** ed. Marvin Kohl, pp. 117–129; Dyck, "The President's Commission for the Study of Ethical Problems in Medicine: Its View of the Right to Life," **Linacre Quarterly** 52 (1985), pp. 110–115.

[47]Gilbert Meilaender, "If This Baby Could Choose . . . " **Linacre Quarterly** 49 (November 1982), pp. 314, 320.

[48]Ramsey, **Ethics at the Edges of Life,** p. 155.

[49]Meilaender, "If This Baby Could Choose . . . " p. 317.

[50]Ibid., p. 318.

[51]Ibid., p. 320.

[52]Eugene F. Diamond, " 'Quality' vs. 'Sanctity' of Life in the Nursery," **America** 135 (December 4, 1976), pp. 396–398; see 398: "The sanctity of life ethic that now spreads its tattered mantle of protection over newborn defective infants must be upheld. It is really protecting all of us." See also: Diamond, "The Deformed Child's Right to Life," in **Death, Dying, and Eu-**

thanasia eds. Horan and Mall, pp. 127–138; Diamond, "The A.M.A. and Infanticide: An Unfortunate Guideline," **Linacre Quarterly** 48 (August 1981), pp. 207–211; Diamond, "Treatment versus Nontreatment for the Handicapped Newborn," in **Infanticide and the Handicapped Newborn,** eds. Horan and Delahoyde, pp. 55–64; Diamond, "A Commentary on the Case of Baby Jane Doe," **Linacre Quarterly** 51 (November 1984), pp. 322–326; Diamond, "Ethical Dilemmas in the Medical and Surgical Treatment of Handicapped Newborns," in **Human Life and Health Care Ethics,** ed. James Bopp, Jr. (Frederick, Md.: University Publications of America, 1985), pp. 191–206; Diamond, "Every Child Should Be Wanted—A Dubious Goal," **Linacre Quarterly** 52 (May 1985), pp. 105–107;

For C. Everett Koop see: C. Everett Koop, "The Sanctity of Life: A Sentiment of the Past?" **Medical World News** 17 (December 1976), p. 112; Koop and Francis A. Schaeffer, **Whatever Happened to the Human Race?** (Old Tappan, N.J.: Fleming H. Revell, 1979); excerpt in **Catholic Digest** 44 (March 1980), pp. 47–49 + ; Koop, "The Silent Domino: Infanticide," **Congressional Record,** 96th Congress 125 (July 17, 1979); Koop, "Infanticide: American Style," **Congressional Record,** 97th Congress 125 (July 18, 1979); Koop, "The Handicapped Child and His Family," **Linacre Quarterly** 48 (February 1981), pp. 23–32; Koop, "The Slide to Auschwitz," reprint ed., **Human Life Review** 8 (Summer 1982), pp. 19–34; Koop, "Interview," **This Week With David Brinkley,** ABC (13 November 1983).

[53]Diamond, " 'Quality' vs. 'Sanctity' of Life in the Nursery," p. 397; Diamond, "Treatment versus Nontreatment," p. 62.

[54]Diamond, "The Deformed Child's Right to Life," p. 136; Diamond, "The A.M.A. and Infanticide," p. 210; Diamond, "Treatment versus Nontreatment," p. 56.

[55]Betty Lou Dotson, "Notice to Health Care Providers,"

Federal Register 47 (June 16, 1982), p. 26027; Also in **Origins** 12 (June 3, 1982).

[56]First revision of Office of Civil Rights of the U.S. Department of Health and Human Services, "Notice to Health Care Providers," including Proposed Rules: Office of the Secretary, DHHS, "Nondiscrimination on the Basis of Handicap Relating to Health Care for Handicapped Infants," **Federal Register** 48 (July 5, 1983), pp. 30846–30852; see also Lawrence Brown, "Civil Rights and Regulatory Wrongs: The Reagan Administration and the Medical Treatment of Handicapped Infants," in **Journal of Health Politics, Policy and Law** 11 (Summer 1986), pp. 231–254.

[57]Second revision: Office of the Secretary, HHS, "Nondiscrimination on the Basis of Handicap Relating to Health Care for Handicapped Infants," **Federal Register** (January 12, 1984), pp. 1622–1654.

[58]Child Abuse Amendments of 1984 [Public Law 98-457] (October 9, 1984); Proposed Regulations to implement statute change: Office of Human Development and Services, Department of Health and Human Services, "Child Abuse and Neglect Prevention and Treatment Program," **Federal Register** 49 (December 10, 1984), pp. 48160–48173; "Final Rule and Model Guidelines for Health Care Providers To Establish Infant Care Review Committees," **Federal Register** 50 (April 15, 1985), pp. 14878–14901.

[59]Ramsey, **The Patient as Person,** pp. 157–164; Ramsey, **Ethics at the Edges of Life,** pp. 160, 212–227; Cahill, "Paul Ramsey: Covenant Fidelity in Medical Ethics," pp. 470–475, esp. pp. 471–475; Cahill, "Within Shouting Distance," pp. 403–407, 412–415; Richard A. McCormick, "Of Death and Dying," in "Notes on Moral Theology, April–September 1972," **Theological Studies** 34 (March 1973), pp. 67–69; also in Richard

McCormick, **Notes on Moral Theology, 1965 Through 1980** (Washington, D.C.: University Press of America, 1981), pp. 437–439; James F. Childress, "Ethical Issues in Death and Dying—Veatch and Ramsey," **Religious Studies Review** 4 (July 1978), p. 186; Veatch, **Death, Dying, and the Biological Revolution**, p. 95; Daniel Maguire, "Correspondence," **Commonweal** (October 6, 1972), pp. 3–4; Donald Evans, "Paul Ramsey on Exceptionless Moral Rules," **American Journal of Jurisprudence** 16 (1971), pp. 184–214.

[60]Ramsey, "Two Concepts of General Rules in Christian Ethics," in **Deeds and Rules in Christian Ethics**, pp. 123–144; Ramsey, "The Case of the Curious Exception," in **Norm and Context in Christian Ethics**, eds. Gene Outka and Paul Ramsey (New York: Charles Scribner's Sons, 1968), pp. 67–135. John Rawls, "Two Concepts of Rules," **Philosophical Review** 64 (January 1955), pp. 3–32.

[61]Ramsey, **Ethics at the Edges of Life**, p. 218.

[62]Ibid., pp. 219, 216; Ramsey, **The Patient as Person**, p. 162; Sherlock, **Preserving Life**, pp. 102–105: Sherlock proposes the lack of "sentience" as a potential cut-off point below which nontreatment is viable.

[63]Helmut Thielicke, "The Doctor as Judge of Who Shall Live and Who Shall Die," in **Who Shall Live?** ed. Kenneth Vaux (Philadelphia: Fortress Press, 1970), pp. 145–194; Hans Jonas, "Philosophical Reflections on Experimenting with Human Subjects," in **Philosophical Essays** (Englewood Cliffs: Prentice-Hall, 1974), pp. 105–131.

[64]Ramsey, **Ethics at the Edges of Life**, p. 213.

[65]MacMillan, "Birth-Defective Infants," p. 624.

[66]Ramsey, **The Patient as Person**, pp. 162–163; Ramsey, **Ethics at the Edges of Life**, p. 216.

[67]Ramsey, **Ethics at the Edges of Life**, p. 215.

[68]Some helpful resources for a fuller treatment of "pain" and "suffering" include: President's Commission, **Deciding to Forego Life-Sustaining Treatment**, pp. 62, 73, 79–80, 277–295; Vincent J. Collins, M.D., "Managing Pain and Prolonging Life," in **New Technologies in Birth and Death** (St. Louis: Pope John XXIII Center, 1980), pp. 144–149; Stanley Hauerwas, with Richard Bondi and David Burrell, "Children, Suffering, and the Skill to Care," in **Truthfulness and Tragedy: Further Investigations in Christian Ethics** (Notre Dame: University of Notre Dame Press, 1977), pp. 147–202. Hauerwas offers a unique, somewhat homiletic treatment of "suffering" and our obligations to care; Maguire, **Death By Choice**, pp. 150–151; Maguire, "Death and the Moral Domain," **The St. Luke's Journal of Theology** 20 (June 1977), pp. 205–206.

[69]Cahill, "Paul Ramsey: Covenant Fidelity," p. 475; A similar critique can be found in Cahill, "Within Shouting Distance," p. 413.

[70]Ramsey, **Ethics at the Edges of Life**, p. 224.

[71]American Academy of Pediatrics, et al., "Principles of Treatment of Disabled Infants," p. 559.

[72]For a fuller critique of Ramsey's theological lacunae see Curran, **Politics, Medicine, and Christian Ethics**, pp. 200–208.

[73]MacMillan, "Birth-Defective Infants," p. 624.

[74]Ramsey, **Ethics at the Edges of Life**, pp. xii–xiii.

[75]Childress, "Ethical Issues in Death and Dying—Veatch and Ramsey," p. 186.

[76]President's Commission, **Deciding to Forego**, p. 26: "Although the Commission has attempted to avoid rhetorical slo-

gans so as to escape the ambiguities and misunderstandings that often accompany them, it uses 'dying' and 'terminally ill' as descriptive terms for certain patients, not as ironclad categories. There seem to be no other terms to use for a patient whose illness is likely to cause death within what is to that person a very short time. Of course, the word 'dying' is in some ways an unilluminating modifier for 'patient'—since life is always a 'terminal' condition—and further refinements, such as 'imminently,' do little to clarify the situation. Therefore, words like 'dying' are used in this Report in their colloquial sense and with a caution against regarding them as a source of precision that is not theirs to bestow."

[77] Ramsey, **The Patient as Person,** p. 133; Ramsey, **Ethics at the Edges of Life,** p. 187. In **The Patient as Person** (p. 63) Ramsey states: "No doubt there are various levels of death (clinical death, physiological death, organ death, cellular death). No doubt also life and death fall within the continuum of all life's processes. . . . No doubt also the individual dies biologically by degrees, and the 'moment' of death is only a useful fiction." It is difficult to imagine that this same Ramsey just eight years later can put such faith in the medical arts to delineate this continuum in physiologically precise terms and then base ethical judgments on those "fictional" distinctions.

[78]Stanley Hauerwas, "Selecting Children to Live or Die: An Ethical Analysis of the Debate Between Dr. Lorber and Dr. Freeman on the Treatment of Meningomyelocele," in **Death, Dying, and Euthanasia,** eds. Horan and Mall, p. 235.

[79]Robert M. Veatch, "The Technical Criteria Fallacy: The Case of Spina Bifida," **Hastings Center Report** 7 (August 1977), p. 15.

[80]Paul R. Johnson, "Selective Nontreatment of Defective

Newborns: An Ethical Analysis," **Linacre Quarterly** 47 (February 1980), p. 43.

[81]Ramsey, **Ethics at the Edges of Life**, p. 155.

[82]Meilaender, "If This Baby Could Choose . . . " p. 317; Lisa Sowle Cahill, "Book Review: **Ethics at the Edges of Life**," **Linacre Quarterly** 46 (February 1979), p. 88; McCormick, "Notes on Moral Theology, 1980," p. 109; John Arras, "Toward An Ethic of Ambiguity," **Hastings Center Report** 14 (April 1984), p. 27.

[83]John R. Connery, S.J. "Prolonging Life: The Duty and Its Limits," **Linacre Quarterly** 47 (May 1980), p. 161.

[84]Ramsey, "In the Matter of Quinlan," in **Ethics at the Edges of Life**, pp. 268–299; Ramsey, "Prolonged Dying: Not Medically Indicated," pp. 14–17.

[85]Richard A. McCormick, "Book Review: **Ethics at the Edges of Life**," **America** 143 (April 8, 1978), p. 289. It should be noted that Ms. Quinlan did in fact die due to such pneumonia-related complications (11 June 1985).

[86]Ramsey, **Ethics at the Edges of Life**, p. xiv.

[87]Cahill, "Paul Ramsey: Covenant Fidelity," p. 475.

[88]Cahill, "Book Review: **Ethics at the Edges of Life**," p. 88.

Chapter Two

A Means-Related Approach to Ordinary/Extraordinary Means

For the past four hundred years, the terms **ordinary** and **extraordinary**, with particular reference to **means** of sustaining life and the effects of those means on given patients, have been an evolving yet fundamental construct in Roman Catholic medical ethics. Given the Church's influence on both culture and scholarship in the West, this concept has spilled over into the wider secular debate concerning the limits, if any, of the generally accepted societal mandate to preserve life. The terms "ordinary" and "extraordinary" actually post-date the sixteenth century introduction of the concepts and content that they have come to symbolize.

Some argue that the concept had its origins three centuries earlier in Thomas Aquinas' attempts to balance one's abiding respect for life with some acknowledgement that the duty to sustain biological life as a temporal good is not absolute. However, it is generally accepted that moral theologians of the sixteenth and seventeenth centuries—e.g., Vitoria, Soto, Banez, Sanchez, Suarez, and DeLugo—formally developed the various elements that distinguish so-called ordinary from extraordinary means. The former, indicating obligatory treatment, has been variously described in terms of usual, natural, simple, available, convenient, and relatively painless or inexpensive. The latter, indicating non-obligatory or optional means, has been associated with treatment procedures deemed heroic, artificial, complex, scarce, inconvenient, excruciatingly painful, or relatively expensive.

The debate continues as to whether the ordinary/extraordinary distinction is one primarily of means objectively analyzed (medical interpretation), or whether it is a more fluid measurement of means in relation to the circumstances and perceptions of a particular patient (ethical interpretation). The President's Commission for the Study of Ethical Problems in Medicine and Biomedical and Behavioral Research devoted thirty pages of its 1983 volume **Deciding to Forego Life-Sustaining Treatment** to the role of such traditional moral distinctions as ordinary/extraordinary and the related notions of acting/omitting and direct/indirect. The Commission concluded that while the ordinary/extraordinary means distinction has moral significance when understood in terms of usefulness (i.e., medical benefit) balanced against burden, its multiple and often ambiguous use across the centuries, as well as the inevitable subjectivity of a given patient's perception of burden, makes any claim "that a treatment is extraordinary more of an expression of the conclusion than a justification for it."[1] It was the Commission's opinion that the ordinary/extraordinary means distinction is too descriptive, too vague, and too subjective to serve as a useful standard for normative ethics.

Is that an accurate assessment? The authors to be incorporated in this chapter, representing a **means-related approach to ordinary/extraordinary means**—Warren Reich, Leonard Weber, John Connery, Donald McCarthy, et al.—would say "no." Acknowledging the prudential dimension of any criterion that attempts to measure the relation of burden to benefit in terms of cost, inconvenience, or pain, these authors see in the ordinary/extraordinary means distinction, rightly understood, a helpful ethical tool. The ordinary/extraordinary means distinction is admittedly in part a results-oriented standard. However, they argue that their approach is grounded in fundamental and abiding principles such that the subsequent situational elements allowed are strictly limited to the direct effects of means used. They contend that this emphasis on means-causation safeguards the inalienable rights associated with the intrinsic worth of every human life.

This chapter will be divided into four sections. As in the previous chapter, we will start with a brief examination of the fundamental presuppositions which undergird the ordinary/extraordinary distinction as it has evolved over the last four centuries. The second section will be a condensed survey of the evolution of the concepts of "ordinary" and "extraordinary" as they have been developed within the Roman Catholic medical ethics tradition. The third section will be the heart of the chapter. What do the contemporary advocates of the ordinary/extraordinary means criterion share in common and how do they differ? The emerging consensus of a means-related ordinary/extraordinary means standard will then be applied to several cases of handicapped newborns to illustrate its practical application. Finally, the chapter will conclude with a critique of the ordinary/extraordinary means standard. What are its strengths and weaknesses both in content and methodology? Is it an effective ethical construct regarding decisions for and against life-sustaining treatment for handicapped infants?

Principles, Presuppositions, A Roman Catholic Ethos

Although the actual terms "Ordinary Means" and "Extraordinary Means" are frequently mentioned in the wider secular debate, scholars who advocate the use of this ethical distinction as the key criterion for decisions concerning life-sustaining treatment are by and large Roman Catholic. A quick survey of Catholic medical ethics manuals of the 1940s and 1950s (McFadden, Kelly, Kenny, Healy) and more recent works (O'Donnell, Ashley-O'Rourke) yields an amazingly parallel set of foundational principles.[2] Five fundamental presuppositions emerge as cornerstones upon which the ordinary/extraordinary means standard builds:

(1) the inherent sanctity or intrinsic worth of every human life;

(2) the inalienable right to life and its preservation;

(3) the principle of Stewardship;

(4) the direct/indirect distinction;

(5) the principle of Totality.

1. As with the medical indications policy previously surveyed, **the inherent worth of every human being** regardless of one's physical or mental capabilities is THE core presupposition. This intrinsic worth is rooted in the Christian belief that every human being is made in the image of God, redeemed in Christ, sanctified by the Spirit, infused with an immortal soul, destined for eternal life, and reflects, by nature, the glory of God. Again and again "official" Roman Catholic pronouncements reflect this core stand in behalf of the intrinsic value of human life.[3]

For the handicapped newborn, and indeed for all disabled persons, this has particular significance. Human worth transcends, or is more deeply etched, than any configuration of biological or mental capabilities. In a decree affirming the United Nations' proclamation of 1981 as an "International Year of Disabled Persons," the Vatican emphasized its defense of "the weak and the suffering."

1. The first principle . . . is that the disabled person (whether the disability be the result of a congenital handicap, chronic illness or accident, or from mental or physical deficiency, and whatever the severity of the disability) is fully a human subject with the corresponding innate, sacred and inviolable

rights. This statement is based upon the firm recognition of the fact that a human being possesses a unique dignity and an independent value from the moment of conception and in every stage of development, whatever his or her physical condition.[4]

This same declaration noted that the quality and moral strength of a society can rightly be measured by the degree of respect and care shown to the weakest, least productive of its members. Accordingly, to devalue anyone because of ill health or handicaps is no less repugnant a form of discrimination than racism, sexism, or any other bigotry. The radical equality of each and all runs deeper than the obvious inequities of human capabilities or personal resources.[5]

2. In the Judaeo-Christian tradition, and even more obviously in the Western philosophical tradition with its emphasis on justice, the inherent worth principle has spawned a corollary, already mentioned above, **the right to life.** University of Chicago ethicist James Gustafson noted that terms like "value," "dignity," and "worth" are not essentially synonyms for "a right."[6] **Dignity** and **worth** merely point to life as a factor that ought to be recognized in decision making calculus. A **right** necessarily implies a pre-eminence or priority for life which lays duty claims on responsible agents. While the embodied "life" of plants and animals calls forth some degree of respect, such generally accepted value does not constitute an unmitigated botanical or animal right to life and its protection. However, it is the assertion of contemporary proponents of the ordinary/extraordinary means distinction, as it was of medical indications advocates, that inherent worth as an embodied member of the **human** species is and ought to be synonymous with rights-bearing status or "personhood." Given the privileged position of humanity in the hierarchy of embodied life, the inherent value of all human lives is further protected by this morally significant "personhood" sta-

tus, implying the rights to life and to equitable access to health care.

3. Inherent worth is linked to the inalienable right to life and to its obligatory protection by a presupposition closely allied to Ramsey's "covenant fidelity" or "canons of loyalty." In a Judaeo-Christian context it is usually referred to as **the principle of Stewardship.** People do not possess their own lives as things to be disposed of at will, but are bound by the living will of the Giver (Dt 22:39; Wis 16:13). The birth of a human infant is perceived as a gift of "life" conferred not only on the individual, but also on all those to whom that person is entrusted for safekeeping and nurture.

Two sorts of obligations emerge with respect to the protection of human life: (1) absolute negative proscriptions and (2) **prima facie,** or **semper but not pro semper,** positive prescriptions. Negatively, all directly willed acts of killing innocent persons are forbidden as fundamental assaults on the intrinsic and abiding goodness of life. In rights language such an absolute negative prohibition safeguards a so-called "immunity right," protecting one's life from all directly intended lethal attacks, whether by commission or omission. Such a presumption absolutely excludes infanticide, however benignly intended, as a fundamental offense against a newborn's life right and presumed best interest.

On the positive side, responsible stewards of life are generally expected to save lives, to enhance biological health and potential, to minimize pain, and, all things being equal, to promote physiological well-being. In rights language the adverb "generally" and the qualifying phrase "all things being equal" imply that there are reasonable limits to this mandate to prolong and sustain "life" in its physiological aspects. Within the Roman Catholic tradition the phrase **semper but not pro semper (always but not for always)** was adopted to indicate that while positive precepts reflect values that must always be revered, other conflicting goods, the limits related to human finitude, and one's commitment to personal and spiritual integrity may, at times, take precedence.[7]

4. This distinction between positive and negative precepts is related to the philosophical **distinction between direct and indirect causation and intention.** Aquinas' explanation of a morally permissible life-taking act of self-defense is frequently cited as a key source for the logic of this distinction. Accordingly, one may never directly intend the death [of the innocent] as the moral species or motive of a lethal act.[8] However, if one's **direct** deed and intention are focused on a defensible human good (e.g., self-defense), then the **indirect** result (the aggressor's death) is regrettably accepted, though unintended, and the agent is morally free of blame. As noted above, all direct infanticide—"direct" deed or "direct" intention of killing even if by omission—is thereby forbidden as an assault on the good of life itself. By contrast, allowing a patient to die, while doing no direct deed and with an intention focused not on killing, but on some good related to the proposed treatment, is seen as morally permissible.

5. Whether one is involved in complex "double effect" cases, in which one's **directly** intended acts of palliative therapy may **indirectly** contribute to suppressed breathing and earlier death, or in more straightforward cases, in which further life-prolongation efforts are judged inordinate to the patient's holistic well-being, the principle of Totality seems to be operative. **The principle of Totality,** elaborated in the 1950s by Pope Pius XII, affirms that in those instances where the relationship of a whole to its parts is operative, "the part is subordinated to the whole and the whole, in its own interest, can dispose of the part."[9] Pius XII's initial referent for this principle seems to have been the human person viewed as a physical organism. In an address to the First International Congress of Histopathology of the Nervous System in September 1952, he developed this

Thomistic notion that the good of the whole person, viewed in terms of bodily integrity, is THE governing factor in medical decisions regarding surgery, repression, or other "mutilation" of one's biological parts or faculties.[10] Logically, the good of the body, on which the worth of the part is ultimately dependent, could in certain cases demand the suppression or removal of a diseased organ.

Is it ever valid to apply the principle of Totality by analogy to an individual more widely considered than bodily integrity? Just as one's organs find their finality in and, in that sense, are subordinate to an effort to sustain one's biological life as a whole, is it ever morally valid "to subordinate" or "to sacrifice" that biological life as a unit for the good of the whole person, in a psychological, social, or spiritual sense? In an address to the International Union Against Cancer (1956), Pius XII seemed to advocate such a possibility: "Before anything else, the doctor should consider the whole man, in the unity of his person, that is to say, not merely his physical condition but his psychological state as well as his spiritual and moral ideals and his place in society."[11]

In the 1950s, prominent Jesuit ethicists Gerald Kelly, John Connery, M. Zalba, and Thomas O'Donnell each interpreted "totality" in this more holistic sense.[12] Pius XII seemed to affirm this broader interpretation of one's totality in a frequently cited 1957 address, "The Preservation of Life."

> A more strict obligation would be too burdensome for most men and would render the attainment of the higher, more important good too difficult. Life, death, all temporal activities are in fact subordinated to spiritual ends.[13]

The following year he stated even more succinctly that "there must be added to the subordination of the individual organs to the organism and its end the subordination of the organism itself to the spiritual end of the person."[14] It is asserted, therefore, that just as organs can be suppressed or even excised for the sake of sustaining one's biological life as a totality, so also prolongation of one's bodily life as a whole need not always dominate in treatment decisions. It can be subordinated, **though not by direct death-intending deeds** (#4 above), to one's psychological, social, and spiritual totality. This is often called the patient's best interest or well-being, holistically considered. The **burden** component of the ordinary/extraordinary means standard seems to operate out of this broader interpretation of Totality, while the question of **benefit** in a strictly medical sense is closer to Pius XII's and Aquinas' original use of Totality in a bodily sense.

In summary fashion the five fundamental principles that undergird the scholars to be surveyed in this chapter are:

1. Every human life has inherent worth (sanctity), regardless of personal potential or handicaps.

2. The inalienable right to life, which involves both the positive **prima facie** obligation to preserve and sustain human life as well as the corresponding negative prohibition against directly intended killing or assault [of the innocent].

3. The principle of Stewardship, by which "life" is seen as a Divine gift, which imposes on its recipient and his/her caretakers duties related to its prolongation and enhancement.

4. The distinction between direct and indirect, with regard to both deed and intention, is posited as a morally significant element in differentiating moral from immoral decisions that result in death. From this distinction emerges the absolute prohibition of all direct killing of innocent life, while allowing for some decisions for nontreatment, which might indirectly,

though unintentionally, contribute to a shortened lifespan.

5. The principle of Totality, which can be explained in one of two life-respecting ways. In the more restricted sense, one's bodily organs find their finality in the "totality" of one's physiological well-being and, therefore, may be subordinated to one's physiological best interest by direct or indirect means. Somewhat analogously, one's biological "life" can be seen as having its ultimate finality in the "totality" of the patient as a biological-psychological-social-spiritual person. While one may never directly negate one's biological life component as one might a diseased organ, one may "subordinate" it indirectly by deeds and intentions focused on one's holistic well-being or best interest.

Ordinary/Extraordinary Means—A Brief Historical Sketch[15]

Most historical surveys of the ordinary/extraordinary distinction begin with a rightful and respectful bow to the writings of the Angelic Doctor, Thomas Aquinas (1225–1274). Later scholars based much of their determination about the general obligation to preserve life and the possible limits to that obligation on Aquinas' concepts of God's dominion over the gift of human life, responsible stewardship, and the positive and negative precepts derived from these.[16] Sixteenth century Dominican moralist Francisco De Vitoria (1486–1546) took up the question of treatment limits with reference to nourishment and to medicinal drugs. In his **Relectiones Theologicae** he dealt with the relationship between a sick person's refusal of food and the potential sinful result, suicide. He concluded that objectively a sick person is obliged to take food for the preservation of bodily life, provided there is some reasonable hope of life. However, if the patient is so depressed that taking food becomes "a kind of impossibility," subjectively speaking, then that patient is not culpable, at least of mortal sin; Vitoria added: "especially if there is little hope of life, or none at all."[17] With reference to kinds or quality of food, Vitoria asserted that one is not required to use the best or most expensive food, even if such foods would be objectively more nutritious.[18]

Building on the premise that one is not obliged to use every possible means, especially if the patient is dying, Vitoria claimed that medicinal drugs are not **per se** obligatory. Nevertheless, if one has "moral certitude" that a particular drug would indeed restore a patient to health, then that drug for that patient becomes, like food, obligatory. Acknowledging that in the state of the sixteenth century medical arts, many medicinal drugs were experimental and questionably effective, the obligation to use them rested on the degree of certitude as to their effectiveness. In dealing with one's obligation to use drugs, Vitoria applied the same cost analysis as he did with "delicate foods." One is not obliged to sacrifice one's whole means of subsistence, nor one's general lifestyle, nor one's homeland in order to acquire a cure or maintain optimum health.[19]

Although Vitoria accepted a patient's particular condition, such as depression, as mitigating one's subjective culpability, he also sought to articulate a more objective standard for discerning potential benefit and what constituted inordinate expense or inconvenience ("a certain impossibility"). He adopted the sixteenth century's version of the "reasonable person" criteria. To fulfill one's positive obligation to sustain life, it is sufficient to perform "that by which regularly a man can live."[20]

Already most of the key components of the later ordinary/ extraordinary distinction are present. Some mention is made of **natural** as opposed to **artificial** means, although Vitoria spoke ambivalently of drugs in both categories. Potential benefit thus seems to be the operative moral component, not naturalness or artificiality. **Reasonable hope of benefit** in terms of a cure or a return to health is a factor in determining obligation, and especially in deciding personal culpability. **Excessive burdens** in terms of financial costs or inconvenience of lifestyle are measured by the **semi-objective standard** of the **common person regularly considered**. Still, **relative factors** related to actual patients in context, such as a patient's personal state of depression, impact both on one's objective obligation as well as on one's subjective culpability for foregoing a procedural means.

Prior to the development of modern anesthesia, surgical procedures not only involved mutilation and disfigurement of the body, but also necessarily involved excruciating pain. Domingo Soto, O.P. (1494–1560) reasoned that surgery, such as the amputation of a limb, because of the inevitable accompanying pain, ought to be categorically optional. Such torture, according to Soto, was beyond the limits that the "common man" ought to be obliged to suffer for one's bodily health. He reasoned that excruciating pain makes an otherwise medically beneficial surgery "morally impossible" to bear.[21] Soto thus added another key component to the tradition of obligatory versus optional means—**excruciating or excessive pain.**

According to studies by Janini and McCarthy, it was Spanish Dominican Domingo Banez (1528–1604) who first introduced the actual terms "ordinary" and "extraordinary" into the discussion concerning obligatory and non-obligatory means for preserving life. Banez upheld the reasonableness of the positive duty to sustain human life, but insisted that one is "not bound to extraordinary means but to common food and clothing, to common medicines, to a certain common and ordinary pain."[22]

The distinction between "ordinary" and "extraordinary" means in all its complexity was explored, summarized, and given synthetic expression in two scholarly articles written by Jesuit moralist Gerald Kelly (1902–1964) for publication in **Theological Studies.** The first article appeared in June 1950. After analyzing the flurry of responses that followed its publication, Kelly refined and revised his definitions of "ordinary" and "extraordinary" means, publishing his final theses in December 1951.[23] In the first article, "The Duty of Using Artificial Means of Preserving Life," Kelly summarized the tradition as represented by the then "standard moralists." He clearly distinguished between the largely descriptive definition of a given means as ordinary or extraordinary and the subsequent moral determination of whether such a means is obligatory or optional.

Ordinary refers to "such things as can be obtained and used without great difficulty," while "everything which involves excessive difficulty" in terms of pain, repugnance, cost, "and so forth" can be labeled **extraordinary.** Reasonably available food, drink, medicines, nursing care, and "most operations and amputations" (given modern anesthesia and therapy) would be **ordinary.** Barring any extenuating or exceptional circumstances, one is morally obliged to seek and use these means to sustain and prolong life. The lone extenuating circumstance which would make such ordinary means optional, even contra-indicated, is if there is no reasonable hope of benefit from the proposed course of treatment, however ordinary in terms of availability and affordability. Kelly noted that he knew of no one who opposes the withholding or withdrawal of means judged useless or futile, which, he suggested, is an application of the axiom **nemo ad inutile tenetur** (no one is held to the useless). At the same time, **extraordinary** means, those in which "excessive" travel, pain, repugnance, or costs are involved, are optional, unless unusual circumstances related to higher duties (the Common Good, prior commitments, or one's salvation) would oblige one to use these still extraordinary means.

In 1950 Kelly was suggesting a two dimensional process for determining whether a proposed medical treatment is morally obligatory: a determination of availability and potential burden under the rubric of ordinary/extraordinary means balanced off against a calculation of the degree of benefit to be derived. For "early Kelly," the question of reasonable benefit is distinct from, but related to the designation of a means as ordinary or extraordinary in terms of burden. The wider genus of obligatory/nonobligatory incorporates both factors.

By the time Gerald Kelly wrote "The Duty to Preserve Life" (December 1951), he had created broader definitions for ordinary and extraordinary means, which were more ethically normative and subsequently have been quoted in most discussions of the ordinary/extraordinary means distinction.

> **Ordinary** means are all medicines, treatments, and operations, which offer a reasonable hope of benefit and which can be obtained and used without excessive expense, pain, or other inconvenience. **Extraordinary** means are all medications, treatments, and operations, which cannot be obtained without excessive expense, pain or other inconvenience, or which, if used, would not offer a reasonable hope of benefit.[24]

The first revision Kelly granted to his critics was that usefulness or reasonable hope of benefit ought to be incorporated into the very definition of ordinary and extraordinary. With his definitions now broadened and clarified, Kelly declared the ordinary/extraordinary means distinction to be morally normative, prescriptive "without qualifications." Ordinary means, those procedures which, as procedures, offer a reasonable degree of medical benefit (therapy) and which are not excessively burdensome, are thereby absolutely obligatory. In contrast, if a procedure offers little or no hope of medical benefit to the patient or, despite potential benefit, if it is excessively burdensome to a given patient, then that means is extraordinary and synonymously optional.

A Means-Related Approach

Whether one chooses to blend reasonable hope of benefit together with a determination of projected personal burden related to the use of a proposed means under the rubric of ordinary/extraordinary means (as "later Kelly" did) or to confine the terms "ordinary" and "extraordinary" solely to the burden component of a wider obligatory/optional calculus (as "early Kelly" did), it is evident that the burden-to-benefit formula proposed here incorporates patient-centered factors that are excluded from the medical indications standard treated earlier. Burden to the patient may in itself override a given patient's obligation to use genuinely therapeutic, even life-saving (i.e., medically indicated) means. If the degree of burden is prudentially judged to be disproportionate to the amount of benefit or degree of health attainable, the patient or one's guardian is free to withhold permission. The principle of Totality is clearly operative in this qualitative preference for "Life" in the fuller sense over against the quantitative prolongation of excessively burdened anatomical functions, "life" in the biological sense.

On November 24, 1957, in an allocution to an International Congress of Anesthesiologists, Pope Pius XII gave clear papal approbation to the ordinary/extraordinary means tradition. Eschewing the determination of what actually constitutes medical death as beyond the Church's competence, he dealt with questions surrounding obligations to resuscitate or to prolong life via artificial respirators. In two brief paragraphs he summarized the key components of the ordinary/extraordinary means distinction as it had been developed since Vitoria.

> Natural reason and Christian morals say that man (and whoever is entrusted with taking care of his fellowman) has the right and the duty in case of serious illness to take the necessary treatment for the preservation of life and health. . . .

But normally one is held to use only ordinary means—according to the circumstances of persons, places, times, and culture—that is to say, means that do not involve any grave burden for oneself or another. A more strict obligation would be too burdensome for most men and would render the attainment of the higher, more important good too difficult. Life, health, and all temporal activities are in fact subordinated to spiritual ends. On the other hand, one is not forbidden to take more than the strictly necessary steps to preserve life and health, as long as he does not fail in some more serious duty.[25]

Contemporary Usage and General Application to Newborns

The ordinary/extraordinary means standard in its contemporary expression is an attempt to ride a middle course between a medical indications policy, which it sees as restricting the patient's right to refuse excessively burdensome means, and a "slippery slope" quality of life ethic, which it sees as jeopardizing an individual's right to life by judging persons as "extraordinary" and expendable as opposed to judging means in relation to given patient-persons.

An extensive survey of the literature yielded four contemporary scholars, all Roman Catholic, who propose and defend the ordinary/extraordinary means distinction as their primary decision-making standard and apply it specifically to the cases of handicapped newborns. Warren T. Reich, Director of the Division of Health and Humanities at Georgetown University's School of Medicine, has published nine articles on the subject.[26] Although he acknowledged that these papers were intended to be the notes "for a thorough essay which never came to the front burner," Reich's unfinished treatment still represents the fullest, clearest, most refined contemporary defense of ordinary/extraordinary means as a normative ethical tool, particularly with regard to the cases of handicapped infants. Leonard Weber, a Director of the Ethical Center at Detroit's Mercy College, published a small volume in 1976, **Who Shall Live?**, subtitled "the dilemma of severely handicapped children and its meaning for other moral questions."[27] In this work, Weber surveyed the positions of four individuals, ultimately endorsing Reich's defense of ordinary/extraordinary means with no significant modifications or criticisms.

If the writings of Drs. Reich and Weber are parallel, so also are the articles defending the ordinary/extraordinary means standard done somewhat collaboratively by two priest-scholars, the late John R. Connery of Loyola in Chicago and Donald G. McCarthy of the Pope John XXIII Center in Braintree, Massachusetts. Convinced that the ordinary/extraordinary means standard is often misinterpreted, Jesuit ethicist John Connery published two nearly identical versions of "Prolonging Life: The Duty and Its Limits" in order to "show that the traditional position, if properly understood, is still a viable one."[28] Likewise, in two parallel articles, written in conjunction with a symposium on **Moral Responsibility in Prolonging Life Decisions,** Donald McCarthy applauds Connery's schema and then attempts to apply it specifically, though quite generally, to the cases of "defective newborns."[29]

The writings of these four scholars will provide the essential content for this survey, with the larger corpus of Warren Reich serving as the thread of continuity. In addition, several other sources—the revised medical ethics "texts" of Ashley-O'Rourke, Haering, and O'Donnell—will be noted in passing as sympathetic to the ordinary/extraordinary means approach. Haering and O'Donnell can be defined as "more or less" advocates, since quality of life components find more open sympathy in their works. The "Vatican Declaration on Euthanasia" (1980) will be presented to determine to what extent this more recent "official" Roman Catholic statement reaffirms Pius XII's approbation of the ordinary/extraordinary means approach. Catholic philosophers Germain Grisez and Joseph Boyle, Jr., openly reject the language of the ordinary/extraordinary tradition, preferring a variation on the "reasonable person" standard. Despite their distinct nuances as to what constitutes a reasonable presumption for or against treatment, it will be argued, in summary fashion, that their reasonable person also operates in accord with the ordinary/extraordinary criteria as presented here.

Reich's explication of the use of ordinary/extraordinary means as a normative decision making standard is most consistently developed in three separate articles published in 1978, two in the **Encyclopedia of Bioethics** and one in a frequently cited anthology on spina bifida edited by Chester Swinyard. Reich and Weber each affirms that there is a normatively binding obligation to accept all "ordinary" means to sustain or prolong life, but there is no strict obligation to use "extraordinary" means. Reich echoes "later Kelly" in defining as extraordinary and optional any life-saving or life-sustaining means that (1) "does not hold out a reasonable hope of medical benefit" or which (2) "also has the effect of causing or perpetuating an excessive hardship" for the patient (and for one's principal caretakers).[30]

By contrast, John Connery rejects this Kelly-inspired movement to incorporate medical benefit into the very definition of what constitutes a means as "ordinary" or "extraordinary." According to Connery, benefit and burden "deal with different issues" and ought to remain distinct. Briefly surveying the tradition he concludes that the hope of benefit component "seems limited largely to terminal cases," while determination of burden is "the decisive factor in the moral distinction" regarding non-terminal patients.[31] In one sense, Connery has merely reinstituted the older language of obligatory/optional for that of ordinary/extraordinary, relegating the latter to one half of the equation, namely "burden" viewed from the patient's perspective.

A Means-Related Approach

Although I tend to agree with Kelly, Reich, and Weber that benefit and burden ought rightly to be conjoined under the rubric of "ordinary" and "extraordinary" means, Connery's preference for the older language is ultimately more a matter of semantics than of actual differences of content. As far as decision making criteria, this chapter combines all who make use of the burden and benefit aspects with reference to specific means, regardless of whether they label the rubric ordinary/extraordinary means, or obligatory/non-obligatory means with ordinary/extraordinary as a subset. The determination of ordinary or extraordinary with reference to a given therapeutic procedure is a sequential process. If the treatment is likely to be successful, **then** this "reasonable hope" of medical benefit must be proportionately weighed against the degree of burden associated with the treatment in order to yield a verdict. However, **if** the treatment is **not** likely to be successful, **then,** regardless of the degree of burden, the non-beneficial means is categorically "extraordinary" and optional.

1. In practice McCarthy, Connery, Reich, and Weber all parallel the medical indications standard in stating that the cases in which treatment is not likely to be successful, offering no reasonable hope of benefit, are "largely" those of so-called imminently dying patients. If "imminently dying" is somehow a medically definable category, then "a life-prolonging procedure which merely prolongs the dying process is considered practically useless."[32] The anencephalic child is the paradigmatic dying infant. Likewise, a certain percentage of myelomeningocele infants (3% by one estimate) are born irretrievably in the dying process. Neither surgery nor medication will appreciably alter this condition or dying process. Therefore, basic nursing care, which one scholar calls "minimal" as distinct from "ordinary" means, is the only generally obligatory prescription.

By the same token, an infant with a better but not ideal prognosis, say for a few months or even a year or two of life,

ought not by that fact alone be left untreated as if handicapped living for that modest but significant span of time is meaningless. Reich offers parameters sufficiently vague enough to allow for prudential case-by-case assessment. If the intended therapeutic treatment "can 'bring the baby through the crisis' to a relatively self-sustaining situation" and if the infant's life can be prolonged "for a not inconsequential period of time" (and "without excessive burden"), then such means are ordinary and obligatory. As Weber sees it, "reasonable benefit" is defined in terms of prolonging life "for a substantial period of time," "a few months" at least or "a year" assuredly. Attempting to define "not inconsequential period of time," Reich refers to Weber and suggests also "perhaps a year."[33]

The prognosis for death in early childhood, such as with Lesch-Nyhan Syndrome or Tay Sachs disease, is not in itself sufficient warrant to declare a procedure extraordinary and optional for lack of benefit. For example, the use of Alopurinol treatments can reasonably benefit Lesch-Nyhan patients, possibly prolonging their life spans, assuredly controlling most non-cerebral symptoms, minimizing the burden. It might be asked how the line of demarcation of "a few months" or "perhaps a year" was established between "imminently dying" and "terminal"? In the former the gain of time is considered negligible and "practically useless," while in the latter it is judged "not inconsequential" and thus generally beneficial and, barring excessive burden, morally compelling. The potential ambiguity of this "dying" category and its use in normative ethics was touched on in the critique section of the previous chapter.

2. What constitutes **excessive burden** and whose hardship can be validly weighed on the scales against potential medical benefit? Reich suggests two categories of excessive burden. If a single procedure or a more prolonged comprehensive treatment viewed as a unit involves excessive pain or risk, it is optional. Or if the mere battle to survive at the same time suppresses "higher

values," such as peace, personal communication, or a loving atmosphere, for a "long period of time," then such a procedure or series would be extraordinary and non-obligatory.[34] In both instances the patient's totality or holistic well-being is allowed to take precedence over mere life-prolongation in a biological sense. Multiple surgeries, lengthy dependence on life-support equipment, prolonged institutionalization, and severe mental or physical handicaps **caused by** the surgery or drugs are listed as some potentially inordinate burdens. Frequently the combination of several of these is a compelling argument for judging a particular means extraordinary.

Reich concedes that excessive hardship may be operative in some of the "more extreme" cases of myelomeningocele infants, for whom years of costly, inconvenient, and potentially painful therapies may yield little proportionate benefit beyond minimal life-prolongation. However, contemporary ordinary/extraordinary means advocates are generally reluctant to delineate further specific burden over benefit scenarios, preferring to give greater weight to potential, even if minimal, benefit in such cases. Donald McCarthy is convinced that instances in which life-prolonging procedures for newborns are extraordinary, and thus optional, in terms of burden-to-benefit ratio, are "infrequent."[35] While noting the theoretical possibility that "excessive" burden might outweigh a reasonable hope of benefit for a given handicapped infant, he offers no case illustrations and immediately presses on to caution against abuses based on "the decision-makers own [presumably biased?] estimate of the value of human life."[36]

Reflecting the inherent worth presumption toward sustaining life, contemporary ordinary/extraordinary means proponents prefer to err on the side of treatment in conflict situations where either the prognosis is unclear or the prediction of burden is, at best, only a "guesstimate." They consider this particularly applicable with reference to infants. The "resiliency" of newborns in terms of both bodily developmental potential and their incredible defiance of prognostic predictability leads Reich to conclude that "there should be a general presumption that pediatric patients have a higher moral claim on 'extraordinary' medical care than do adult or elderly patients."[37] While this might inappropriately be read as a quality of life bias for youthfulness over maturity, in fact it bespeaks a medically-accepted circumstantial component that tips the benefit/burden scales, in the case of children, toward greater potential bodily healing for the risks involved. In addition to the medically indicated better odds for success, infants at the beginning edge of life have more "life" to lose, at least quantitatively speaking, by a premature decision to forego or cease treatments.

It might be suggested that the language of "extraordinary" means is used somewhat inconsistently here. If we elect to use costly, inconvenient, or relatively painful measures, which is presumably what is meant by "extraordinary" in this instance, because children are more likely to respond and in fact heal (defying usual prognosis), does not the procedure suggested thereby become "ordinary" because of its benefit over burden proportion? Is not the delineation of it as "extraordinary" merely a premature or hypothetical **descriptive** judgment? **Normatively**-speaking, wouldn't it be more accurate to Kelly's 1951 definitions of "ordinary" and "extraordinary" to say that pediatric patients are more likely, due to bodily resiliency and the tenuousness of neonatal prognoses, to benefit from treatments that in an older patient **might be** deemed excessively burdensome and "extraordinary"? So for infants, such admittedly burdensome treatments are frequently not disproportionate to the potential benefit and thus can be labeled situationally "ordinary" and generally obligatory.

John Connery defends this presumption for treatment by emphasizing that extraordinary means implies "optional," but that "optional" is **not** a synonym for "ought not use." In the case of handicapped persons, particularly infants at the dawn of life, proxies ought not too rashly judge that this patient would prefer nontreatment. Such a presumption is often biased by a quality of life prejudice that a life lived with such handicaps as retardation, paralysis, or the loss of some important faculty is horrible, unbearable, "a life not worth living." No statistical evidence exists indicating that disabled persons are any more prone to suicide than people with more "ideal" physiques or IQs. No hard data suggests that they would generally choose non-life rather than handicapped existence.[38] In short, Connery suggests that reasonable persons, handicapped or otherwise, generally accept **some** extraordinary risk, pain, cost or inconvenience in an effort to sustain life and gain a modicum of good health. Parents or guardians acting on behalf of handicapped infants ought to decide for them with this same "reasonable person" presumption. Extraordinary means implies the option **to use** as well as **to refuse.**

Up to this point we have concentrated on medical benefit and the degree of burden **for the infant.** Indeed this is appropriate since the patient's best interest is and ought to be the principal focus of parents and health care professionals. However, the patient is not an isolated subject, but is also a social being, a member of the commonweal. As such a competent patient or a non-competent patient's proxy may rightly factor familial and social concerns into the determination of means-related excessive burden. Pius XII included "grave burden for oneself or another" in his definition of extraordinary means.[39] The degree of hardship incurred by the family in caring for a handicapped infant is not inconsequential. Excessive emotional or financial strain on parents and fellow siblings is a genuine component of an infant's life situation. With sufficient caution against potential greed, selfish motives, or parental guilt, contemporary ordinary/extraordinary means proponents allow the category of burden to include some room for familial costs related to proposed courses of treatment.[40]

If the responsibility for care "overtaxes" the financial or psychic resources of the infant's family, threatening the "essential functioning" of that family unit, perhaps their obligation to be the providers of such ordinary care has been exceeded. In a sense, what is "ordinary" in terms of the infant's individualistic needs becomes "extraordinary" for his/her family to provide. Reich refuses to see such familial claims and needs as a "right" to be set over against a newborn's inherent "right" to be alive. No one, particularly in a family context, has a "right" to be free from all serious hardship or the rightful claims of loved ones. Practically speaking, however, there are cases in which exorbitant financial costs of prolonged treatment and perhaps the emotional drain on personal resources so tax a family that it becomes a "moral impossibility" for them to continue as the sole providers for a handicapped infant's cure and care.

Reluctant to delineate when such a critical juncture is reached, Reich notes that the society at large still retains its **parens patriae** obligation if the treatment is truly ordinary from that infant's perspective. The next logical question is: Could the long term costs of a handicapped infant's medical treatments and care ever be judged excessively burdensome even for society, and therefore categorically extraordinary and optional? Weber firmly rejects this possibility in the present practical sphere. "We do not recognize any circumstances where the very treatment of a child would impose an intolerable burden upon society."[41] If anything, the true character of a society is made manifest in the effort it expends for its least productive, most needy members. Reich, on the other hand, implies that "**every** possible form of lifesaving treatment, even the most expensive, for all diseased and defective infants" may be considered an excessive burden on society's finite resources and complex demands for equitable macroallocation or distribution.[42] Dominicans Benedict Ashley and Kevin O'Rourke suggest that theoretically, if beneficial means prove excessively burdensome or even unjustly taxing to a family's or a society's finite resources, the wartime principle of triage might be applied to determine who "deserves" the available resources.[43]

In summary, (1) if an infant is clearly dying, that is when death is irreversibly coming within minutes, hours, days or a few weeks at most, all therapeutic means or life-sustaining devices cease to be medically beneficial and are relatively useless. Such means are judged extraordinary and optional. Taking into account the burden of such means on the infant and one's care-takers for minimal or no useful purpose, one might read "optional" as "ought not use." Minimal means or nursing care, within the limits of "do no harm" medical practice, are indicated. (2) If the patient is not dying and a proposed means will be of some even minimal therapeutic benefit, the presumption is toward treatment unless burdens **related specifically to the use of such means** are judged excessive for the child or, in a patient-oriented sense, for one's family unit. Generally the State takes over financial and support responsibility for the handicapped patient's care if "burden" exceeds parental limits. (3) Finally, given the infant's being at the beginning edge of life and a child's statistical potential for defying negative prognoses, parents and health care professionals ought not equate "generally" extraordinary means (excessive burden with risky or minimal benefit potential) which are optional, with a presumption for non-use. Even these generally burdensome means, in the case of resilient newborns, may be situationally ordinary and more or less clearly indicated for use.

It is important to note that the burden of being handicapped prior to and not caused by the proposed treatment is generally **inadmissible** in this burden/benefit calculus. According to contemporary proponents of the ordinary/extraordinary means distinction, the quality of the patient's life unrelated to means causation ought not be allowed to impact on decisions made to accept or forego medically beneficial and manageably burdensome treatments. The burden-to-benefit proportionalism of the ordinary/extraordinary means tradition admits that quality of life elements impact on the **prima facie** presumption for treatment. It would be historically inaccurate to suggest that the extraordinary means concept referred to means qua means, whereas contemporary quality of life ethics speak more to the extraordinary condition or quality of the patient's life. As Reich expressed it,

> . . . the "extraordinary means" concept was never concerned about the means themselves, but about whether the **qualitative** aspects (pain, hardship, futility of the treatment, the extremely adverse condition of the survivor) of the **use** of some medical or other life-support effort might in a given **situation** diminish the obligation to treat.[44]

For Reich, Weber, Connery, and McCarthy the limiting factor is that the quality of life, which, if judged to be excessively burdensome, can make the presumably beneficial treatment extraordinary and optional, must be caused by or directly related to the use of the means contemplated. In other words, "the burden must be the burden of a medical treatment, not the burden of a handicapped existence."[45] If a suggested therapeutic procedure, such as radical surgery or prolonged chemotherapy, causes excessive fear or repugnance **before,** is extremely painful **during,** or leaves one gravely inconvenienced and inhibited **after,** then, and only then, does one have the right to weigh that burden against potential benefit.[46] In answer to the question "Why are quality of life considerations allowed if they are related to the use of the means and not apart from such a relationship?" John Connery succinctly responds:

A Means-Related Approach

> When a person is afflicted with some handicap through no
> act or fault of his own, he certainly deserves sympathy, but
> he does not bring the handicap on himself. It is because a
> moral choice is involved in decisions regarding means to pro-
> long life that related burdens become pertinent.[47]

Accordingly, one is never obligated to choose life-prolonging means which directly cause or contribute to an excessively
burdened life or which directly inhibit to a substantial degree
one's experience and pursuit of psychological, social, or spiritual
well-being, "Life" in its totality. To forego or withdraw such excessively burdensome treatment as extraordinary is to choose
how to live one's life qualitatively over against merely prolonging
it quantitatively. In no sense is this a direct attack, either by deed
or by intention, on the inherent value of life in its physiological
aspects. One is making a decision "for" the patient's well-being,
not "against" the good of "life" in its temporality. However, it is
argued that incorporation of one's fundamental, albeit tragic
handicap into the ethical equation, except where such data im-
pacts on the reasonableness of the benefit or the "copeability"
of the patient to deal with burdens accompanying treatment, is
to directly declare some lives in themselves as lesser, unequal,
not worth saving. This, according to contemporary ordinary/ex-
traordinary means proponents, is blatantly prejudicial against
the inherent and equal dignity of all human beings and an injustice against the infant patient's rights to life and equitable access to available health care.

In practice, contemporary ordinary/extraordinary means
proponents see such a bias operative in the various "Babies Doe"
court cases, in which the presence of one handicap has influenced decisions regarding other **largely unrelated** medical
problems. According to the twofold criteria of benefit and burden surveyed here, treatment would seem obligatory for a
Down's Syndrome baby with digestive blockage (the Hopkins

111

and Bloomington Cases). Since surgery offers reasonable hope of success, and the burden of the surgery for the patient would not normally be excessive, the surgery itself cannot be regarded as extraordinary.[48] While living with a handicap such as Down's Syndrome is less than ideal and may even be a real cross to bear for the patient and family, such a condition in this case is not a burden related to or caused by the means. The fact that an infant is physically or mentally handicapped should not **in itself** be considered a reason to withhold treatment, but is legitimate only to the extent that such disabilities impact on the medical feasibility or level of burden of a proposed new course of treatment.

It is appropriate here to mention two borderline cases—Ramsey's Curious Exceptions—which admittedly are not dealt with at length by any of the authors surveyed. (1) Is the case of a **permanently unconscious but non-dying infant** one in which therapeutic means could be deemed relatively useless, extraordinary, and optional? (2) Is the case of an **infant in irremediable pain** one in which the burden is so excessive that all therapeutic means, however beneficial, should cease and aggressive palliative care begin? In an attempt to defend the possible withholding of treatment from the permanently comatose patient, philosophers Germain Grisez and Joseph Boyle suggest that in point of fact most permanently unconscious patients "can be presumed to be dying."[49] The cause of the comatose state already at work in the person will most likely be the eventual cause of death. If so, then such mentally deficient or severely brain-damaged infants fall within the "dying" category noted above, for whom all treatment is relatively non-beneficial, and rightfully they demand only minimal means and care. However, if the "few months" or "one year" time limit cited by Weber and Reich has any bearing on the definition of "dying," some permanently unconscious infants live longer, defying inclusion under the dying-therefore-don't-treat category.

Connery seems to be speaking of somewhat similar cases of

severely brain deficient infants when he allows that "there may be a rare case where predictable quality-of-life would be so low that the life itself could not be classified as human. . . . "[50] Most such infants are mercifully born already dying. However, if such an issue from the womb survives, Connery seems on thin ice (the "monstrosity" mindset of a former era) to deny human status to living human bodies no matter how deformed or deficient.

If an infant is in intractable pain, either physical or the less definable area of mental anguish, palliative relief seems to be humane and mandatory. If a proposed therapeutic means causes or prolongs irremediable suffering, by definition such a procedure is excessively burdensome, optional, even contra-indicated. If the pain persists even without the procedure, the principle of Double Effect, which is rooted in the direct/indirect distinction, allows ordinary/extraordinary means proponents to administer up to and including potentially lethal doses of morphine or other palliative drugs, provided the **direct** deed and intention are the administration of pain medication to alleviate suffering, **not** the death of the child as such. According to these ordinary/extraordinary means proponents direct infanticide is **always** a violation of the infant's inherent dignity and life right. However, indirect "allowing to die" is morally defensible **either** when further therapies would be medically useless and/or excessively burdensome **or,** in this instance, when direct attempts to relieve pain indirectly suppress respiration even to the point of shortening one's life and/or dying process.

"Sanctity of Life" vs. "Quality of Life"— A Methodological Strawperson

Reich asserts that the debate between so-called Sanctity of Life positions, such as the ordinary/extraordinary means standard or the Medical Indications policy of Paul Ramsey, and the so-called Quality of Life positions, in which projected abilities and patient potential unrelated to means causation play a key role, is principally one of ethical methodologies. The former he labels "traditional deontological positions," while the latter he gathers under the heading of "consequentialism." A roughly parallel methodological dualism is set up by Leonard Weber under the headings "classical ethical worldview" versus "modern ethical worldview."[51] In his 1974 Testimony before a Senate Subcommittee on Health, Reich labeled the methodology underlying Quality of Life criteria as an "ethic of outcomes." By contrast he suggested that a sounder and safer approach would be an "ethic of rights," anchoring his Sanctity of Life presumption in a deontological (i.e., duty-oriented) base.

Despite disclaimers by both Reich and Weber asserting that such a dualistic polarization of actual scholars into two mutually exclusive methodological camps bespeaks only an "artificial construct," they proceed in analyses to portray all quality of life ethicists as utilitarians, espousing a purely "consequentialist calculus." It is "as if" all proponents of a quality of life standard (unrestricted to means causation) deny the inherent values which undergird the so-called Sanctity of Life position—the dignity and equality of every human life.[52] Reich and Weber continue to speak of their position "as if" it is somehow deontologically pure, duty-based sans consequences.

This dichotomizing of methodologies into only two mutually exclusive possibilities is neither an accurate portrayal of the method employed by most ordinary/extraordinary means advocates, who are too facilely labeled "deontologists," nor a fair characterization of some of those advocating the admission of quality of life factors. In their endeavor to differentiate the ordinary/extraordinary means tradition from an ethic which admits quality of life factors not restricted to the use of means, Reich and Weber too sharply define the methodological battle lines. It is fair to say that contemporary ordinary/extraordinary means proponents, and the Roman Catholic medical ethics tradition in general, have operated from a more principle-bound ethical model, one which espouses inherent worth, rights, and corresponding natural duties. However, in terms of norms and decision making, particularly with reference to the burden dimension of the ordinary/extraordinary means standard, the method is more results-oriented or consequentialistic than Reich or Weber seem to admit. Likewise, to caricature all quality of life proponents as if they are pure utilitarians or consequentialists is inaccurate, a bit polemical, and unfair. Such a presumed dichotomy or polarization does a disservice both to the consequentialism of application present in the ordinary/extraordinary means tradition as well as to the **prima facie** right-making rules espoused by many, though not all, quality of life proponents.

Other Ordinary/Extraordinary Means Sympathizers

To complete this section it is appropriate to briefly mention the writings of four theologians, two philosophers, and one Church document which tend to affirm the ordinary/extraordinary means standard. The revised and variously updated medical ethics "texts" of Benedict Ashley with Kevin O'Rourke, Bernard Haering, and Thomas J. O'Donnell all reflect the general lines of the ordinary/extraordinary means standard. Dominicans Ashley and O'Rourke devote only four pages of their lengthy volume **Health Care Ethics** to the ordinary/extraordinary means distinction. Immediately they note the confusion between a medically descriptive use of the terms "ordinary" and "extraordinary," as often used by physicians, and their ethically normative use by moralists, which "takes into consideration the total situation of the patient, the nonmedical, as well as the medical factors." After a sketchy survey and citation of Kelly, Pius XII, and the Vatican's 1980 "Statement on Euthanasia," Ashley and O'Rourke conclude that "the practical difficulties in applying" the ordinary/extraordinary means distinction, especially in cases involving discontinuing a means already utilized, "will always remain." In their 1986 second revision of this text, Ashley and O'Rourke downplay the language of ordinary and extraordinary, while retaining its basic content.[53]

Respected Redemptorist theologian Bernard Haering, while advocating the core content of the ordinary/extraordinary means distinction, and while denouncing quality of life arguments for euthanasia as "contemptuous" and "a dangerous application of Darwin's theory of the survival of the fittest," at the same time suggests a shift in terminology to "beneficial/non-beneficial" and himself acknowledges the inevitable and rightful presence of some quality of expected life components in decisions concerning non-dying patients.[54] Haering briefly mentions three types of cases—those in which the patient is imminently and irreversibly dying, those in which medical treatment will offer "some hope to restore health or at least . . . tolerable life," and those in which the illness is incurable or terminal in a long range sense. In the first instance, it is reasonable to withhold or withdraw a treatment that is "not at all beneficial" from a "child who is doomed to die." In the case of reasonably curable patients, beneficial treatment seems morally obligatory. The validity of incorporating quality of life factors associated with or caused by given means is upheld by Haering, though he declines to emphasize the causal linkage as plainly as Connery's analysis.

> Most experts in medical ethics would, certainly, allow the patient to refuse an intervention that probably might be life-saving but reduce his life to extreme misery.[55]

Apparently a "miserable" quality of life brought about by the potentially life-saving intervention is sufficient grounds to warrant refusal of such "means." Positively stated, if there is a well-grounded or even a faint hope that treatment will yield a "rea-

sonably happy" and "significant existence" for a short (not defined) or longer period of time, then such means ought to be
employed.[56] The echoes of Reich and Weber are obvious.

Jesuit Thomas J. O'Donnell, both in his medical ethics texts
and in his contributions to **The Medical-Moral Newsletter,** has
highlighted two features of the ordinary/extraordinary means
tradition. The first is that "one cannot, for the most part, speak
of therapies and techniques as **simply** ordinary or extraordinary,
but only **relatively** so, i.e., relative to the total mental, moral and
physical condition and prognosis of the patient."[57] The second
is his advocacy of the term "minimal means" for hospice-like,
non-medically beneficial care that is generally obligatory for
dying and incurable patients. This is to differentiate it from "ordinary means," which more accurately refers to obligatory medical or therapeutic care. Quality of life advocate Richard
McCormick sees in O'Donnell's "relativity" an acknowledgment
that the burden/benefit ratio is not restricted to effects directly
caused by means, but reflects more widely " . . . the relation of
a due proportion between the cost and effort required to preserve this fundamental context [for other goods], and the potentialities of the other goods that still remain to be worked out
within that context [life itself]."[58] O'Donnell responded that he
and McCormick are in basic agreement, and yet he balked at
adopting the language of "quality of life" because of the potential abuse to which such a standard lends itself.[59]

In the decades since Pius XII has the Roman Catholic
Church made any formal pronouncements on the ordinary/ex-
traordinary means standard? The June 1980 "Vatican Declaration on Euthanasia," adopted by the Sacred Congregation for
the Doctrine of the Faith and approved by John Paul II, mentions but does not categorically endorse the ordinary/extraordi-
nary means tradition. While unequivocally reaffirming the
tradition's condemnation of euthanasia as "an offense against the
dignity of the human person" and a "crime against life," the doc-

ument treats the ordinary/extraordinary distinction more ambiguously.

> In the past moralists replied that one is never obliged to use "extraordinary" means. This reply, which as a principle still holds good, is perhaps less clear today by reason of the imprecision of the term and the rapid progress made in the treatment of sickness. Thus some people prefer to speak of "proportionate" and "disproportionate" means.[60]

Acknowledging both the ambiguity of language and the ever advancing medical technology with regard to prolonging vital signs even as brain activity may ebb away to stem-only functioning, the Vatican grants some recognition at least to the language of proportionalism. Is this a step toward acceptance of some projected quality of life factors unrelated to means into the ethical equation? Or is the Sacred Congregation limiting such considerations to those strictly related to means, as contemporary ordinary/extraordinary means proponents defend?

> In any case, it will be possible to make a correct judgment as to the **means** by studying the **type of treatment** to be used, **its** degree of complexity or risk, **its** cost and the possibility of using **it**, and comparing these elements with the result that can be expected, taking into account the state of the sick person and his or her physical and moral resources. [my emphases]

At present "official" Roman Catholic spokespersons seem not to push the burden elements beyond those related to the type of treatment or means considered for use. At most, the "Vatican Declaration on Euthanasia" can be seen as consistent with and in no way contradicting the ordinary/extraordinary means standard surveyed in this chapter. Opponents and revisionists of the ordinary/extraordinary means standard, particularly those advocating a broader use of quality of life elements and a so-called proportionalist methodology, see in the document an openness, a possible first step toward their position and method.[61]

Before moving to the critique section, it is appropriate to mention briefly the pertinent writings of two Catholic moral philosophers, Germain Grisez and Joseph Boyle, Jr.[62] In their joint volume, **Life and Death with Liberty and Justice**, Grisez and Boyle adopt a "reasonable person" standard as the best safeguard against selfish and/or arbitrary decisions to withhold or withdraw treatment based on some "unjustifiable discrimination" against the non-competent or handicapped.

> The basic requirement of justice with respect to care for noncompetent persons is easy enough to state: The noncompetent person ought not be denied that care which any reasonable person who was competent probably would desire in similar circumstances, and the noncompetent person ought not be given care which any reasonable person would refuse in a like case.[63]

In terms of specific case applications, Boyle's emphasis here and elsewhere on "the character of the treatment" and their joint exposition of "the ordinary standard of due care" parallel closely the nontreatment exceptions espoused by those labeled proponents of the means-related approach to ordinary/extraordinary means. They assert that reasonably "anyone would refuse experimental treatments," which are defined as "those with a minimal chance of success and those which would prolong the dying process without giving at least some increased opportunity for action."

Grisez and Boyle propose a three pronged ethical-legal guideline for determining reasonableness with reference to treatment of handicapped infants:

1) In the case of so-called dying infants, parents in consultation with the physician may reasonably and therefore morally withhold or withdraw treatment.

2) If the infant is not irreversibly dying, and if surgery or treatment will in fact sustain life and improve future potential, then parental decisions for treatment are ethically reasonable and should go unchallenged.

3) If the patient is not dying, but is in such a wretched, painful, or relatively incurable state that costly and aggressive treatment may be judged excessively burdensome to the patient or to others, then parental and physician consensus to withhold or withdraw medical treatment may be reasonable, but not conclusively so.[64]

As Boyle sees it, making decisions to withhold or withdraw treatment solely with the intention of avoiding the burdens of the treatment is no species of injustice.[65] What Grisez and Boyle seek to categorically exclude is any judgment that is based on the quality of the patient's life itself. So, while they reject the language of "ordinary" and "extraordinary," their version of a "reasonable person" thinks and operates quite comfortably within the traditional ordinary/extraordinary parameters.

In summary, means-related ordinary/extraordinary means proponents, like Reich, Weber, Connery, McCarthy, et al., espouse a decision making standard which rejects both the reduction of a patient's best interest solely to medical benefit as well as all conscious determinations that "kinds" or "qualities" of life **in themselves** exclude patient-persons from access to care. As Leonard Weber sums it up:

Perhaps the real value of the extraordinary means approach is, then, that it puts the whole question in the context of the goodness of life and of our obligation to respect that goodness. . . .

First, it does not accept actual killing. . . . When dealing with infants who cannot contribute to the decision of whether to treat or not, this emphasis on the inherent goodness prevents parents or others from assuming that "they have full and prior dominion over the life of the newborn."

Secondly, the emphasis on the nature and consequences of the means used provides for some protection against an arbitrary decision being made on the basis of a judgment about the worth of a particular type of life.[66]

Means-Related Approach to Ordinary/Extraordinary Means: A Critique

The ordinary/extraordinary means standard, the oldest and in some sense the most developed of the formal positions to be surveyed in this volume, has much to commend it for normative use. Grounded in many of the same fundamental presuppositions and values as the medical indications policy, it nonetheless is more open to contextualizing the value of biological benefit or mere life-prolongation within the broader context of the totality of the patient. Its proponents acknowledge that the quality of one's life in terms of burden, albeit related to means causation, is rightful grist for determining a handicapped infant's holistic best interest. In that sense, unlike the medical indications standard, the ordinary/extraordinary means tradition takes into account the fuller psychological, social, and spiritual components of a patient-person's well-being, whether s/he is imminently dying, terminal in a long-term sense, or not dying at all. Incorporation of the burden element as a counter-balance to biological benefit or mere life prolongation in the cases of "non-dying" patients is the genius of the ordinary/extraordinary tradition.

As with the medical indications policy, this author does not disagree with any of those cases which ordinary/extraordinary means proponents accept as optional candidates for nontreatment. Rather, I question whether there might not be others for whom nontreatment is also in their best interest, whose life conditions themselves are excessively burdened, prescinding from and irrespective of means causation. Therefore, while this critique will to a large extent be a positive affirmation of the major components of the ordinary/extraordinary means tradition, ultimately the standard will be rejected as a normative tool more for its ambiguities and inadequacies than for any blatant error.

As noted in the previous chapter this researcher accepts the need for fundamental values and presuppositions. With that in mind, I am generally in agreement with four of the five presuppositions set forth as underpinnings for the ordinary/extraordinary means tradition. (1) Belief in the inherent worth or dignity of human life is core, the necessary presupposition for all ethics, for all discussion of human freedom, justice, obligations, and limits. While some debate could ensue among the various disciplines as to when the product of conception is or becomes human, it is generally accepted that a live-born issue from a woman's womb is a person, a rights-bearing being worthy of respect. (2) I also uphold the principle of Stewardship. Life is a gift, entrusted to us for safekeeping and growth, not a possession to be used, abused, or disposed of at will. In a special way parents, guardians, and society are entrusted as "caretakers" of all voiceless, helpless non-competents, particularly newborns at the beginning edge of life. (3) I espouse the principle of Totality, both in the wider sense of holistic integrity as well as in the narrower sense of bodily wholeness. The inclusion of psychological hardship and patient-centered familial and social factors indicate that this more holistic sense of a patient's totality or best interest is operative in the burden-to-benefit proportionalism of the ordinary/extraordinary means tradition. (4) Likewise, the positive duty to preserve, promote, and prolong human life is a fundamental obligation of communal living. Stewardship, justice, and Gospel love each calls forth this personal and social **prima facie** duty. The language of rights and corresponding duties is frequently used to express a given patient's claim on such care.

(5) The final fundamental presupposition, rooted in the valid **descriptive** distinction between direct and indirect, is the negative and presumably absolute proscription of all direct killing of innocent human life. The direct/indirect distinction and the related double effect principle are commendable historical attempts to preserve life and limit morally licit killing, lest a "slippery slope" to euthanasia on demand ensue. However, the stress on directness or indirectness of the act itself, the questions surrounding the meaning(s) of moral intention, and the reluctance in the tradition to link human acts together into wider spheres have led a number of scholars on the "left" and "right" to question the act-centeredness of the absolute prohibition of all direct killing of innocent life as well as the usefulness of the double effect principle itself.

These criticisms lead some revisionists, both proportionalists and theory of compromise advocates, to question the **absoluteness** of this precept.[67] In pastoral practice, the use of a revised Double Effect methodology (Grisez, Boyle, et al.) and the application of proportionalism (McCormick, Knauer, et al.) often yield the same conclusion, as in the case of the removal of an ectopic fetus. Since the focus of this volume is the criteria for nontreatment decisions, not the subsequent question of direct infanticide, further delving into the direct/indirect controversy would be tangential from our stated purposes here. One need not do nor intend "killing," either by commission or by omission, to defend nontreatment of some severely handicapped newborns based solely on the quality of life they are destined to live post-treatment.

In addition to its fundamental principles, the contemporary ordinary/extraordinary means standard is to be commended both for its patient-centeredness and for its fuller or more dynamic interpretation of the patient's well-being. Patient-centeredness is here contrasted with a social utilitarianism, in which individuals are valued or expendable depending on corporate usefulness and productivity. Focusing on each patient's best interest, contemporary ordinary/extraordinary means proponents reflect the best of the Roman Catholic social tradition of the last century. "Common good" has consistently been seen as inextricably linked to the well-being and flourishing of each individual, **not** as some socialistic subjugation of individuals to the society.[68] The meaning of "patient's best interest" in the ordinary/extraordinary means tradition admirably bespeaks a fuller sense of one's well-being, in which the physiological aspects of life may be overridden or indirectly subordinated as one chooses to enhance other, arguably "higher" aspects of human flourishing.

I believe that inclusion of **burden** as well as **benefit, proportionately weighed,** is core content and method for any ethically complete determination of treatment versus nontreatment. Acceptance of the principle of Totality means that one's physiological benefit ought to always be seen in the wider context of one's burdens, ability to cope, and total best interest. What constitutes a valid burden, whether the condition of one's life itself unrelated to means can be such an excessive burden, and how much is enough benefit to warrant treatment—these rightly remain debatable questions, open to logical analysis and judgment. The "relativity" of general case applications and the "subjectivity" of ultimate patient culpability rightly indicate that treatment decisions are prudential, defying textbook precision.

Finally, I agree with the following case applications made by means-related ordinary/extraordinary means advocates: Further therapeutic treatment of anencephalic or other "imminently dying" infants is futile and potentially cruel, thus unwarranted. Failure to treat a potentially life-threatening condition, such as digestive blockage, based on the presence of another anomaly of the caliber of Trisomy 21 (Down's Syndrome), would be prejudicial and generally immoral. Trisomy 21 in itself is an insufficient burden to the child or to one's family to warrant nontreatment. I would concur with contemporary ordinary/extraordinary means proponents in preferring to err on the side of treatment and life wherever "potential" benefit or "borderline" excessive burden is present. After all, some generically "extraordinary" means, as noted by Reich and McCarthy, may be more potentially useful and "ordinary" in the case of resilient newborns.

Despite this appreciation for the presuppositions, components, and general application of the contemporary ordinary/extraordinary means standard, ultimately its shortcomings outweigh its strengths as a normative tool. I propose two substantive objections and one caution to the use of this distinction as a decision making standard: (1) multi-layered ambiguity of definitions; (2) overemphasis on the importance of the "related to means" restriction; and, (3) in the case of handicapped infants, a potential for undercutting the patient's right via proxy to judge burdens excessive and a treatment optional.

1. However descriptively valid the burden-to-benefit content of the ordinary/extraordinary means standard may be, the ambiguity of definitions and multiple uses of the same terms tend to frustrate rather than foster its use as a normative ethical tool.

> . . . you do not need to puzzle for very long over the categorical distinction between 'ordinary' and 'extraordinary' means of saving life. By that I mean those terms as classes or categories of treatment are no longer useful.[69]

The President's Commission, most critics of the ordinary/extraordinary means distinction, and even to some degree the Vatican "Statement on Euthanasia" concur with Paul Ramsey's assessment. "Confusion," "inherently unclear," "vague and ambiguous," "imprecision of the terms," "dangerously deceptive appearance of simplicity," and "surrounded by ambiguities" are some of the phrases used to characterize the misconceptions that surround the very definition of the terms **ordinary** and **extraordinary**.[70] Ramsey and others have noted the distinction between the "descriptive" use of the terms by medical professionals and the fuller, more value-laden "prescriptive" use of the language of ordinary and extraordinary by moralists.[71] For a physician, procedures which are fairly common, available, and standard in current medical practice are labeled "ordinary" regardless of patient factors, by contrast with unusual, scarce, and experimental treatment options, which are descriptively "extraordinary." Ethicists bring to bear the patient's diagnosis, prognosis, personal and social situation, and right to refuse excessively burdensome therapies, transforming a description of means qua means into an obviously more comprehensive trans-biological, morally determinative discussion of the quality of a patient's life related to the use of means. Frequently, health care professionals and ethicists misunderstand each other when using the terms ordinary and extraordinary. Speaking about "means" being ordinary or extraordinary is inherently though unintentionally misleading, since ethicists, who coined the distinction in the first place, are not primarily talking about medical procedures or means as such. They are making qualitative judgments about a patient's medical prognosis and degree of burden in defining a **situation** as ordinary or extraordinary.

Nor is this confusion about whether "ordinary" and "extraordinary" refer to means or to situations involving proposed means restricted neatly to the misunderstanding between physicians and ethicists. Even within the moral literature scholars frequently confuse, overlap, and intermingle the descriptive and prescriptive uses of the terms. To help clarify the meaning of **ordinary** and **extraordinary** within the tradition one can point out at least four distinct layers or "meanings" that are used, even at times within the same ethical article:

a. "Ordinary" and "Extraordinary" can refer in some largely objective sense to the distinction between means, as procedures in themselves, which are natural as compared with those that are artificial. Reflecting Vitoria's ambiguity concerning the "naturalness" or not of medicinal drugs, Kelly likewise used some unstated criterion for declaring some drugs natural and "ordinary," while others, like insulin, remained artificial and "extraordinary." The natural/artificial distinction in itself seems to be never morally absolute. So-called artificial means, such as synthetic drugs, respirators, or radical surgery, are judged ethically not on the basis of some arbitrary determination of "naturalness," but on the degree to which they are beneficial and/or burdensome to the patient.

However, Kelly seems to have resurrected the natural/artificial distinction to suggest that purely natural means, what today are frequently called "basic care" by contrast with "curative procedures," are always "ordinary" and obligatory. Disagreements concerning what constitutes basic or natural care were left unresolved by Kelly.[72] Artificial means, defined in this instance as all therapeutic procedures, serious surgeries, or chemical substances, are in themselves ethically neutral. Potential benefit and/or burden are the morally determinative factors.

b. "Ordinary" and "Extraordinary" can refer to the distinction between procedures qua procedures that are usual and/or available versus unusual and/or scarce based on some semi-objective determination of standard medical practice within a given culture and era. This, as noted above, is often described as the medical or physician's use of the terms. Is this a morally significant distinction? The most accurate answer is "sometimes." If the procedure is extremely risky and experimental or if it simply is unavailable in one's region, then it is "physically impossible" or at least questionably beneficial for use. In this case **descrip-**

tively extraordinary is equivalent to **morally** non-obligatory. However, common and available, as connotations for ordinary, do not in themselves constitute a means morally obligatory.

c. "Ordinary" and "Extraordinary" can be used to refer not so much to the procedures in themselves but to the effects those procedures have on patients **in general.** Here is Vitoria's "man regularly considered" criterion, which is generically objective, but morally non-absolute. Roman Catholic manualists of the 1940s and 1950s attempted to clarify what the then current measurable definitions of "excessive" pain, cost, and inconvenience were **for the average person.**[73] Such components as pain, cost, and inconvenience are objectifiable by third parties only hypothetically, and these estimates are of little ultimate value in actual moral determination. As Kelly noted, determination of "excessive" burden is relative to a particular patient's own experience and circumstances, not morally objectifiable in an a priori sense. Nonetheless, some ethicists in the tradition brought to bear a reasonable, though unproven principle that no one ought to be obliged to spend or endure more cost or pain than some admittedly generic norm—e.g., Healy's $2,000 surgery limit in 1956 or Soto's assertion that surgery pre-anesthesia ought to be categorically optional.

d. "Ordinary" and "Extraordinary" are also used as the terms to describe the effect a treatment has on a given patient in terms of his/her unique circumstances and personal experience of varying "degrees" of pain, cost, or inconvenience. The tradition has ultimately let this level be THE moral determiner of obligation or non-obligation.

If "ordinary" and "extraordinary" are used for all four types of distinctions, then confusion and a conflictual use of terms seems inevitable. For example, serious surgery would be an **extraordinary** means in terms of its being artificial; **ordinary** in terms of it being commonly used and available in contemporary medical practice; still **ordinary** in terms of it being generally affordable (with insurance coverage) and relatively painless; and ultimately it could be **extraordinary** based on excessive cost, pain, inconvenience, or repugnance to a given patient. The equation of "extraordinary" with optional would be inapplicable at level one, applicable only if extraordinary at level two, inapplicable at the "rule of thumb" level, and really only morally determinative at the subjective or personal level four.

This ambiguity as to the precise meaning of "ordinary" and "extraordinary" continues among contemporary proponents. Two examples will suffice. John Connery asserts that "only the patient can gauge the burden of his experience." Consequently a means subjectively deemed excessively burdensome is by definition "extraordinary" and morally optional **for this patient.** How then can Connery at one point conclude that such procedures as giving oxygen, IV feeding, and blood transfusions "might have been considered extraordinary means 50 or a hundred years ago," but today, except in some isolated third world countries, they are presumably ordinary, thus obligatory.[74] Does Connery mean "ordinary" and "extraordinary" in terms of formerly unusual or scarce procedures now being convenient and relatively inexpensive? If so, then he has allowed the so-called descriptive and generic meaning of "ordinary" and "extraordinary" to hold sway, while the subsequent determination of burden to a particular patient seems, in this instance, already to be excluded from his labeling of means as obligatory or optional.

The second example of possible ambiguity of terms comes from two of Warren Reich's 1973 sources and parallels Connery's desire to objectively define at least some means as "ordinary" de facto, regardless of circumstantial burden or benefit. According to Reich, " . . . we are always obliged to employ ordinary means to preserve life, even in hopeless cases," or, in another source, "even if there is no real hope of recovery."[75] If a case is hopeless, with no real possibility of recovery, would not

all means thereby be non-beneficial and by (later Kelly's) definition be "extraordinary" and optional? Are there such obligatory "ordinary" means qua means that defy inclusion in the burden-to-benefit calculus?

Jesuit scholar Thomas O'Donnell offers a possible solution by differentiating **curatively** beneficial, reasonably non-burdensome **therapeutic means** from **non-curative,** albeit humanely beneficial and non-burdensome **care** for a dying or terminal patient. The former constitute "ordinary means" within Kelly's normative definitions, while the latter, being non-beneficial in a medical or healing sense, O'Donnell labels "minimal means."[76] To avoid terminological overlap and confusion these "minimal means" ought not be called "ordinary" and yet, like ordinary means, they are obligatory. He defines "minimal means" as "basic sustaining and hygienic measures, such as normal feeding, resting and other usual assistance (such as clearing the air passages of the newborn)."[77] Pius XII, Kelly, Reich, Weber, Connery, et al. acknowledge this obligation to continue hospice-like care even after all curative or therapeutic means prove useless or excessively burdensome.

Some well-publicized neonatal court cases indicate that even "normal feeding" may at times be "contra-indicated." An esophageal fistula or a duodenal atresia renders normal digestion impossible. Prior to corrective surgery, normal feeding of such infants would be potentially fatal. In short, it seems that even O'Donnell's "minimal means" are not absolute, but rightly fall back within the domain of relatively "ordinary" and "extraordinary" means, depending upon circumstances and prognosis, as well as patient "copeability." Although a caring intention ought always to be obligatory, delineating specific acts in themselves as always the caring thing to do and thus obligatory is questionable. The right of some patients in some circumstances to refuse even basic nourishment dates back to Vitoria, the founding scholar of the ordinary/extraordinary means tradition.

The introduction of the idea of so-called "ordinary" or minimal means that are obligatory even when hope of benefit is nill only serves to further the ambiguity of terminology. As Ramsey rightly noted, the language of ordinary and extraordinary is "incurably circular until filled with concrete descriptive meaning."[78] That "descriptive meaning" is not limited to a physician's estimate of benefit percentages nor a reasonable person's presumption of cost, pain, or repugnance thresholds. Ultimately, as the President's Commission concluded, determination of a means in context as extraordinary "is more of an expression of the conclusion than a justification for it." Gary Atkinson concluded his survey of the ordinary/extraordinary means tradition prior to Pius XII with the thesis that Kelly's 1950 to 1951 shift from a more descriptive use of the terms to a more normative and inclusive use serves more to confuse than to clarify the ethical issues.[79] Attempts since Kelly to use the terms prescriptively flounder in the same definitional overlap and imprecision.

2. Laying aside the false dichotomizing of Sanctity of Life versus Quality of Life positions, which gives a mistaken impression of categorical methodological distinctions, means-related ordinary/extraordinary means proponents ultimately acknowledge the quality of life dimensions inevitable in judging "reasonableness" with reference to relatively beneficial or life-sustaining means and "excessive" with reference to patient burden. By transcending the physician's and the reasonable person's interpretations of means judged largely in themselves, contemporary ordinary/extraordinary means proponents admit that it is not the means as such which are labeled "ordinary" or "extraordinary," but the means as they enhance or inhibit a given patient's quality of life or total well-being, including biological as well as psychological, social, and spiritual interests.

Thus, a proposed course of treatment which indeed could save a life (e.g., surgery on a duodenal atresia) or would prolong life indefinitely (e.g., respirator-assisted breathing) is not "ordinary" or "extraordinary" as a means save in the circumstantial context of a given patient. Both of these procedures could be judged relatively "extraordinary" for an infant with anencephaly or in the latter stages of Lesch-Nyhan syndrome. However, to withhold either from an infant whose only other anomaly is Trisomy 21, particularly if the level of retardation is prognostically mild, or whose "premie"-related respiratory distress will likely be temporary, is judged by many as a species of discriminatory bias. Such means would seem to be "ordinary" and obligatory in these cases. Is it really the means that ought to be labeled "ordinary" or "extraordinary" in these scenarios or is it not more accurate to say that the means objectively are "ordinary"—beneficial and relatively burden-free? Rather, would it not be more accurate to say that it is the patient's quality of life with or without the proposed means which is judged "ordinary," that is curable and manageably handicapped, or "extraordinary," that is hopeless or excessively burdened? Indeed, **causation** of burden **by the use of means** may, in some cases, be the key component in the moral determination of ordinary obligation or extraordinary license. However, it is questionable whether "caused by" or "related to" means is as morally determinative as contemporary ordinary/extraordinary means proponents imply.

The ordinary/extraordinary tradition, at its best, allows patients to take into account one's pre-procedural state—dying, severe retardation, myelomeningocele, deafness, cancer, quadraplegia—in determining whether a means will cause an added burden, tipping the scales from tragic but tolerable to excessive, thus making the proposed procedure optional due to the patient's extraordinary projected state post-treatment.[80] For example, the loss of eyesight through some life-sustaining brain surgery would not usually be considered an intolerable burden for an otherwise healthy patient. However, if the patient is already deaf, mute, and quadraplegic, then the burden of these "other" pre-surgical factors are not and ought not be excluded from the determination of how burdensome sightless life will be for this specific patient. The patient's unique situation is always an essential component in determining the morality of use or non-use. Even if a given means will indeed cure the disease or save the organ, the patient is not reducible to his disease or her organ.[81] One of the beauties of the ordinary/extraordinary means tradition has been that it is patient-oriented, not disease-centered.

If the burden of pre-means handicaps plus the burden "caused by" proposed means can be tallied to equal a quality of life or a state of well-being that is extraordinarily burdensome to the patient, why is it not valid to tally a pre-means state that is judged **already** extraordinarily burdensome plus a proposed means judged relatively neutral, beneficial to prolonging "life" in its physiological aspects, but ultimately not beneficial to one's holistic well-being, to reach the same excessive burden judgment and option for non-use? After all, the burden-to-benefit ratio is not of a means related to organs functioning, but of a means related to one's total situation, "pre-" as well as "post-" treatment.

Kennedy Institute founder, the late Dr. Andre Hellegers, broached this topic in a brief but insightful article entitled "What Is 'Extraordinary' in Maintaining Life?"[82] Written against the backdrop of the famous Johns Hopkins case, Hellegers posed two cases of possible treatment refusal clearly within the ordinary/extraordinary means tradition. In each case the proposed "means" is massive brain surgery to remove a malignant tumor. In the first case, prior to surgery the patient tells the physician not to proceed if it becomes clear that **all** of the malignancy cannot be removed. As the patient said, "I don't want half my brain removed needlessly. I would rather die normally than to spend another month paralyzed, blind, and unable to think." This is an open and shut case of a patient determining that the burden of life with half a brain removed is excessive for the minimal benefit of so brief an extension of life. One might declare such non-curative, minimal life-prolongation relatively useless or hopeless. The situation would be judged **extraordinary** and the proposed radical surgery **optional.**

In the second case the prognosis is not terminal, provided the tumor covering a similarly large portion of the brain is removed. Again, the patient refers to the post-surgery probability of paralysis, blindness, and the inability to think "for the rest of my days" as sufficient burden to declare the post-surgery state **extraordinary** and the admittedly beneficial surgery **optional.** As the patient pleaded, "It would ruin my family and I simply could not stand being a vegetable." Psychic pain, repugnance, and familial burden are all classic components of the ordinary/extraordinary means distinction.

Hellegers then offered a third case, that of a patient who is severely retarded **prior** to the proposed life-saving means. The proposed necessary surgery is the relatively routine removal of a duodenal atresia. Failure to correct this intestinal problem would prohibit digestion, thus leading to starvation if not fed or death by choking if fed naturally. Prescinding from the question of personal versus proxy consent, the major variation between this case and the famous Hopkins case is that Hellegers posited a specific and extreme mental diagnosis and prognosis—an IQ of 30 as well as paralysis, blindness, and the permanent inability to think. Hellegers asked,

> If it is permissible for a man to forego a brain operation which leaves him with an IQ of 30, may he [or his proxy] forego an operation on his duodenum which leaves him with an IQ of 30?

He readily acknowledged the difference that in the former cases the operation caused the mental deficiencies and loss of faculties, while in the latter case they existed independent of and prior to the proposed surgery. Hellegers challenged,

> But I would ask whether the repugnance is at what **causes** the state or at what it **results** in. I submit it is the result we act on.

Foregoing any in-depth analysis of what definitively would constitute an excessively burdened life, he wondered if the decision to forego life-saving brain surgery based on a determination that post-surgical burdens will be excessive is really so ethically distinct from a decision to forego duodenal surgery based on a similar determination. In the end Hellegers questioned if the determination of excessive burden in the cases of non-dying patients is morally restricted to those "caused by" or "directly associated with" the means used. He concluded,

> Perhaps classic ethical categories like "extraordinary means" are not adequate to the task of analyzing such (non-terminal) cases.[83]

In short, must the means actually cause the burden that one judges extraordinary or can one forego means that are morally neutral in themselves based on a determination that their use will prolong an **already** "extraordinary" and inordinately burdened life? Just as the so-called "imminently dying" state pre-means is sufficient to declare all contemplated means, however minimally beneficial, as useless and/or excessively burdensome, is it not possible to project some extremely wretched state of handicapped existence that is so "useless" **to the patient** or so "burdensome" **to the patient** that any proposed means for any related or independent ailments would only serve to perpetuate the burden needlessly?

In his article in the Swinyard anthology, Reich attempted

to incorporate such neutral means into the widest possible definition of extraordinary means. In addition to those inordinate burdens "directly associated with" or "caused by" the use of proposed means, Reich concludes that even if excessively burdensome qualities are merely "perpetuated by" life-sustaining treatment, such means can be labeled "extraordinary" and their use becomes optional, perhaps even contra-indicated. According to Reich,

> This category . . . would include some infants afflicted with meningomyelocele and other newborn anomalies. As regards those infants who can be expected to experience at least a minimal self-consciousness and freedom of will and who therefore will be striving to achieve moral (or moral-religious) self-realization, the duty to preserve life may be limited by the excessive hardship that would forseeably be experienced by the patient if his entire striving to discover moral meaning in life were to be totally submerged in or utterly strained by the mere effort to survive and by the suffering that accompanies that effort.[84]

If life post-treatment will be solely or excessively bound up in the effort to keep biological functions operative with little or no practical potential for further (or perhaps any) "moral self-realization," then such treatment would seem **optional** based on the **extraordinary** life situation of the patient, regardless of whether the means cause the tragic condition or merely "perpetuate" it. Apparently, Reich is suggesting that a mere life-sustaining therapy, which serves only to perpetuate an excessively burdened, experientially-deprived life, can be seen as indirectly causing or in some sense contributing to the extraordinary situation of the patient. In that sense the perpetuating means can be judged extraordinary and mercifully optional.

Reich is absolutely correct in his conclusions, but perhaps stretches the notion of "means-related" too far in declaring the judgment about foregoing such life-sustainers to be about **means** in any causal or meaningful sense. Weighing the use of obviously life-sustaining, arguably painfree devices for a patient whose whole conscious effort would be caught up or "submerged" in that life-prolonging effort, it may be more correct to say for this patient that nothing substantial, no personal good save metabolism is to be gained by prolonging treatment. His/her quality of life **irrespective of means contemplated** is "extraordinary." S/he has become the exception to the **semper** but not **pro semper** obligation to preserve life. "Perpetuated by" is so passive, so intransitive a verb form as to make the linkage between the means involved and the decision for nontreatment to be morally irrelevant.

If a newborn is "permanently unconscious" or in a "chronic vegetative state" due to pre-natal or neonatal oxygen deprivation, the value of drug therapies, ventilator assistance, or surgery for relatively unrelated problems (all generically "ordinary" means) may rightly be foregone in the name of the patient's extraordinarily burdened quality of life or reasonably hopeless prognosis for much in the way of human flourishing, participation in life's "higher goods." In terms of such a non-dying patient's total best interest, the decision to forego further therapies is in no real sense contingent on judgments about the means, but about the patient's tragic condition **prior to** and **irrespective of** means-related data.

On the other hand, if the infant is only mildly retarded, as with Down's Syndrome, or a case of hydrocephalus diagnosed and shunted early, then the relative value of those same procedures comes into play because the quality of life or potential well-being of such a patient, while imperfect and in some sense regrettable, is in no way so burdensome nor so hopeless that s/he is exempt from the obligation to preserve life. Since such children are capable of participating in the transbiological dimensions of human flourishing and personal fulfillment, it is in their embodied best interest to be saved, cured, and/or sustained. It is the patient's quality of life with or without means which is the focus of the nontreatment decision. If the means impact on the patient's experience of life, qualitatively-speaking, then "related to means" is a valid moral factor. However, even when means are in some tragic cases relatively insignificant, the patient's qualitative experience of burden vis-à-vis benefit is still THE core operative criterion.

The "means restriction" of the contemporary ordinary/extraordinary means standard serves more as a wedge to forestall decisions for direct infanticide, a sort of second line of defense if the direct/indirect distinction crumbles, than it does as an accurate reflection of the actual content of the standard with reference to nontreatment questions. The very question of treatment versus nontreatment implies that a proposed **means** is on the board for discussion. Still the decision to use such therapy or mere life-sustaining devices is not necessarily related to the **means** itself at all. Underlying **every** decision for nontreatment is a decision about the quality of and potential for the patient's well-being, whether means affect, detract, or remain neutral to that determination.

3. The third and final criticism is more of a caution or a potential danger. The preference for the use of so-called "extraordinary means" in the case of infants, as advocated by all four of our major authors, if pushed too far, undermines the infant's fundamental right, through parents or proxy, to judge a means excessively burdensome, regardless of potential curative or medical benefit. In their understandable desire to minimize potential bias or injustice by parents, Reich, Weber, Connery, and McCarthy may inadvertently be bordering on a medical indications policy, which tends to undercut a patient's freedom and right to be the primary arbiter and interpreter for self of burden-to-benefit proportionalism. The wisdom of the ordinary/extraordinary means tradition is threefold:

a. Parents, in consultation with the medical team, have a right, in the patient's behalf, to opt for usually or descriptively "extraordinary" means based on a minimally hopeful prognosis and the unpredictability of neonatal resilience.

b. Society has a right, in the patient's behalf, to challenge potential bias against a handicapped infant by parents or health care agencies, thus forestalling injustice.

c. However, the beauty of the ordinary/extraordinary tradition is that decision making is **not** restricted to determination of benefit in a medical sense. Parents, in consultation with competent professionals, and always in the infant's best interest, have the right as proxies to withhold or withdraw even potentially beneficial treatment based on a determination of **excessive burden** for the patient (and for others). This dimension ought not be curtailed, lest non-dying infants be forced to endure **all** treatment in the name of possible benefit, negating the "burden" component altogether, thereby truncating the holistic best interest or totality of the neonatal patient-person.

Conclusion

From Vitoria to Reich or Kelly to Connery, the value of human life, patient-centeredness, respect for an agent's responsible freedom, potential medical benefit, and the possible validity of excessive burden proportionately outweighing that biological benefit have been core content for any truly ethical decisions to treat or not to treat. As a **description** of the complexity of the nontreatment decision making process, the various elements of the ordinary/extraordinary tradition rightly expand one's perspective beyond the narrowly focused medical indications approach. However, as a **normative** method or a **prescriptive** process for practical application it is inadequate—vague and ambiguous in terms of language and too bound to "means causation" to allow for the quality of life judgments necessary in tragic cases of excessive burden or hopeless life-prolongation unrelated to means. Determinations about means qua means, such as scarcity, usualness, and generic usefulness, have been indiscriminately intermingled with determinations not necessarily related to means, such as a patient's qualitative judgment of "reasonable" benefit or "excessive" burden. Incorporating the relative elements of a patient's prognosis and circumstances and subjective interpretations into the equation and then declaring the means as "ordinary" or "extraordinary" gives a potentially misleading impression of objectivity and means-centeredness.

> The distinction between ordinary means and extraordinary means has a dangerously deceptive appearance of simplicity. It appears to be a distinction made by assessing means of treatment, whereas in fact . . . 'the criteria for decision relate primarily to the patient not to the remedy.'[85]

Once one moves beyond a descriptive determination of whether a proposed procedure is available, reasonably safe, and therapeutic as opposed to experimentally risky, determination of "ordinary" and "extraordinary" as moral categories is largely not a question of means at all, but of the patient's quality of life "with" as opposed to "without" treatment. Proponents of a medical indications policy see this "quality-of-life ingredient" as a dangerous tilt toward patient autonomy and subjective voluntarism. On the other hand, admitted quality of life advocates see the ethical task as one neither of eliminating quality of life projections nor of limiting them to those caused directly by means. Rather, the task is to create general parameters or definitions of "meaningful" versus "excessively burdensome" life conditions or qualities within one's religious or philosophical framework. To the extent that proposed means impact on or cause burden or benefit, they are factors to be reckoned with. To the extent that a proposed means, especially one which merely sustains metabolic functions, neither enhances nor inhibits one's wider well-being, decisions to continue or to cease such means would seem to be more basically quality of life judgments irrespective of means.

NOTES

[1]President's Commission, **Deciding to Forego,** pp. 82–90.

[2]Charles McFadden, O.S.A., **Medical Ethics for Nurses,** (Philadelphia: F.A. Davis, 1946). Revised five times under the title **Medical Ethics** (Philadelphia: F.A. Davis, 1949, 1953, 1956, 1961, 1967); Gerald A. Kelly, S.J., **Medical-Moral Problems** (St. Louis: Catholic Hospital Association of the United States and Canada, 1958). Compilation of five booklets, published 1949–1954; John P. Kenny, O.P., **Principles of Medical Ethics** (Westminster, Md.: Newman Press, 1952, 1962); Edwin Healy, S.J., **Medical Ethics** (Chicago: Loyola University Press, 1956); Thomas O'Donnell, S.J., **Morals in Medicine** (Westminster, Md.: Newman Press, 1956, 1959). Revised under the title **Medicine and Christian Morality** (New York: Alba House, 1976); Benedict M. Ashley, O.P. and Kevin D. O'Rourke, O.P., **Health Care Ethics: A Theological Analysis** (St. Louis: The Catholic Hospital [Health] Association, 1978, 1982); revised again as **Ethics of Health Care** (1986).

In addition to these textbooks, the following overviews of Roman Catholic medical ethics survey the principles covered in this section: Charles E. Curran, "Roman Catholicism," in **Encyclopedia of Bioethics,** ed. Warren T. Reich (New York: The Free Press, 1978), pp. 1522–1534, esp. pp. 1528–1529; Robert M. Veatch, **A Theory of Medical Ethics** (New York: Basic Books, 1981), pp. 33–40; Bernard Haering, **Medical Ethics** (Notre Dame: Fides Publishers, 1973), Ch. 6, pp. 65–115, esp.

pp. 65–75; David F. Kelly, **The Emergence of Roman Catholic Medical Ethics in North America** (Lewiston, N.Y.: Edwin Mellen Press, 1979).

[3]John Paul II, **Familiaris Consortio** (12/15/1981) (Washington, D.C.: USCC Publications, 1982), number 30; Congregation for the Doctrine of the Faith, "Vatican Declaration on Euthanasia," **Origins** 10 (August 14, 1980), pp. 154–157; National Conference of Catholic Bishops, **Human Life in Our Day, A Pastoral Letter** (11/15/1968) (Washington, D.C.: USCC Publications, 1968); Vatican Council II, **Gaudium et Spes**, in **The Documents of Vatican II**, ed. Walter M. Abbott, S.J. (New York: Guild Press, 1966), pp. 199–308, esp. numbers 12, 27; John XXIII, **Pacem in Terris** (4/11/1963), in **Renewing the Earth**, eds. David J. O'Brien and Thomas A. Shannon (Garden City, N.Y.: Image Books, 1977), pp. 124–170, esp. numbers 9–10.

[4]Vatican Statement, "The International Year of Disabled Persons," **Origins** 10 (May 5, 1981), p. 747.

[5]Ibid., p. 748; Protestant ethicist Stanley Hauerwas bases his "Ethic of Care" on this point. Ethical decisions with reference to the weak and handicapped, particularly infants, say more about our values as moral agents than about the potential medical benefits and burdens to the non-competent patient. See Hauerwas, Bondi, and Burrell, "Children, Suffering and the Skill to Care," in **Truthfulness and Tragedy**, pp. 147–184.

[6]James M. Gustafson, "Commentary on Daniel Callahan's 'The Sanctity of Life,'" in **Updating Life and Death**, ed. Donald R. Cutler (Boston: Beacon Press, 1969), p. 232.

[7]Daniel A. Cronin, **The Moral Law in Regard to the Ordinary and Extraordinary Means of Conserving Life** (Rome: Typis Pontificiae Universitatis Gregorianae, 1958), p. 43. In this

section Cronin cites Fanfani and Lehmkuhl as his authorities for the distinction between positive and negative precepts.

[8]Thomas Aquinas, **Summa Theologica**, II, II, q. 64, a. 7–8. Some controversy centers around Aquinas' alternate cases of capital punishment meted out to criminals and the willful destruction of military enemies in wartime. Did St. Thomas allow one to "intend" death as the moral species of the act in these cases? Without pausing to solve this debate, it is clear that he did absolutely outlaw directly intended life-taking of "innocent" persons, which, obviously, all newborns are.

[9]Pius XII, "Address to the First International Congress of Histopathology of the Nervous System" (September 13, 1952), **The Pope Speaks** (1952), p. 106.

[10]Ibid., pp. 98–107; excerpted and discussed more fully in Martin Nolan, "The Principle of Totality in Moral Theology," in **Absolutes in Moral Theology?** ed. Charles E. Curren (Westport, Conn.: Greenwood Press, 1968), pp. 232–248.

[11]Pius XII, "Cancer, A Medical and Social Problem," p. 48, as cited in Lisa Sowle Cahill, "A Natural Law Reconsideration of Infanticide," **Linacre Quarterly** 44 (February 1977), p. 50.

[12]Gerald Kelly, "Pope Pius XII and the Principle of Totality," **Theological Studies** 16 (1958), p. 379; John R. Connery, S.J., "Current Theology: Notes on Moral Theology," **Theological Studies** 15 (1954), p. 602; E. Regatillo-M. Zalba, **Theologiae moralis summa II** (Madrid: Biblioteca de Auctores Cristianos, 1953), n. 251; Thomas J. O'Donnell, S.J., **Morals in Medicine,** pp. 71–72.

[13]Pius XII, "Prolongation of Life," **The Pope Speaks** 4 (1958), pp. 395–396. Nine months earlier Pius XII addressed similar issues in a "Speech to the Italian Anesthesiological Society," **The Pope Speaks** 2 (1955/1956), pp. 33ff.

[14]Pius XII, "Tranquilizers and Christian Morals," **The Pope Speaks** 5 (1958/1959), pp. 8–9.

[15]Daniel A. Cronin, **The Moral Law in Regard to the Ordinary and Extraordinary Means of Conserving Life** (Rome: Typis Pontificiae Universitatis Gregorianae, 1958); Jose Janini, "La operation quirurgica, remedio ordinario," **Revista Espanola de Teologia** 18 (1958), pp. 331–348; James J. McCartney, "The Development of the Doctrine of Ordinary and Extraordinary Means of Preserving Life in Catholic Moral Theology Before the Karen Quinlan Case," **Linacre Quarterly** 47 (August 1980), pp. 215–224; Gary M. Atkinson, "Theological History of Catholic Teaching on Prolonging Life," in **Moral Responsibility in Prolonging Life Decisions,** eds. Donald G. McCarthy and Albert S. Moraczewski (St. Louis: Pope John XXIII Center, 1981), pp. 95–115.

[16]Thomas Aquinas, **Super Epistolas S. Pauli** (Taurini-Romae: Marietti, 1953), II Thessalonians, Lectio II, n. 77; Thomas Aquinas, **Summa Theologica,** eds. Anthony Ross, O.P. and P.G. Walsh, Blackfriars Ed. (New York: McGraw-Hill, 1966), II, II, q. 126, a. 1 and ad. 3; On Suicide: II, II, q. 64, a. 5; On Killing the Innocent: II, II, q. 64, a. 6; On Self Defense: II, II, q. 64, a. 7 and 8; On Mutilation: II, II, q. 65, a. 1.

[17]Francisco De Vitoria, **Relectiones Theologicae** (Lugdini, 1587), Relectio IX, de Temp. n. 1. " . . . maxime ubi est exigua spes vitae aut nulla." Taken from Cronin, p. 49.

[18]De Vitoria, ibid., n. 12; De Vitoria, **Comentarios a la Secunda Secundae de Santo Thomas** (Salamanca: Edition de Heredia, 1952), II, IIae, Question 147, article 1.

[19]De Vitoria, **Relectiones Theologicae** Relection. IX, de Temp. n. 9 and 12.

[20]Francisco De Vitoria, ibid., n. 1. " . . . satis est, quod det operam, per quam homo regulariter potest vivere."

[21]Domingo Soto, **De Iustitia et Iure** (Venice, 1568), Lib. 5, Question 2, article 1; Referred to in John R. Connery, S.J., "Prolonging Life," p. 153; McCartney, "The Development of the Doctrine," p. 216; Janini, "La operation quirurgica," p. 333; Cronin, **The Moral Law in Regard,** p. 51.

[22]Domingo Banez, **Scholastica Commentaria in partem Angelici Doctoris S. Thomae** (Duaci, 1614–1615), Tom. IV, **Decisiones de lure et Iustitia, II,** IIae, Question 65, article 1; referred to in Cronin, **The Moral Law in Regard,** p. 47; Janini, "La operation quirurgica," pp. 335–336; McCartney, "The Development of the Doctrine," p. 216.

[23]Gerald Kelly, S.J., "The Duty of Using Artificial Means of Preserving Life," **Theological Studies** 11 (June 1950), pp. 203–220; Gerald Kelly, S.J., "The Duty to Preserve Life," **Theological Studies** 12 (December 1951), pp. 550–556.

[24]Gerald Kelly, S.J., "The Duty to Preserve Life," p. 550. With the addition of the phrase "for the patient" in line three, Kelly reasserts the same definitions in his 1958 text **Medico-Moral Problems** (St. Louis: Catholic Hospital Association of the United States and Canada, 1958), p. 129.

[25]Pius XII, "Prolongation of Life," pp. 395–396.

[26]Warren T. Reich, "On the Birth of a Severely Handicapped Infant," **Hastings Center Report** 3 (September 1973), pp. 10–11; Reich, "Testimony" (6/11/1974), Hearing before the Subcommittee on Health of the Committee on Labor and Public Welfare, United States Senate. Examination of the Moral and Ethical Problems Faced with the Agonizing Decisions of Life and Death, 93rd Congress, 2d session, 11 June 1974, pp. 53–62;

Reich, "What Rights Have the Newborn?" **Origins** (July 4, 1974), pp. 89–91; Kenneth Guentert and Warren T. Reich, "Should We Let That Child Die?" **U.S. Catholic** 40 (October 1975), pp. 6–13; Reich, "Quality of Life and Defective Newborn Children: An Ethical Analysis," in **Decision-making and the Defective Newborn,** ed. Chester A. Swinyard, pp. 489–511; Reich, "Life: The Quality of Life," in **Encyclopedia of Bioethics** (New York: The Free Press, 1978), pp. 829–840; Reich and David E. Ost, "Infants: Ethical Perspectives on the Care of Infants," in **Encyclopedia of Bioethics,** pp. 724–735; Reich and David E. Ost, "Infants: Public Policy and Procedural Questions," in **Encyclopedia of Bioethics,** pp. 735–742. David Ost's contributions to the field seem limited to these two articles done in collaboration with Dr. Reich; Reich, "Preferential Education in Policies for the Handicapped," **Momentum** 12 (May 1981), pp. 16–19; Warren T. Reich, "On Sustaining the Lives of Defective Newborn Children" McMath Lecture (October 15, 1973); Reich, "Defective Newborn Children: An Inquiry into 'Quality of Life' Ethics." Skytop, Pa. Conference (May 4–6, 1976). These unpublished studies became the bases for Reich's **Encyclopedia of Bioethics** entries; Reich, "Value of Life in the Theological Perspective of Karl Rahner," A.A.R. Symposium on Rahner (November 21, 1978).

[27]Leonard J. Weber, **Who Shall Live? The Dilemma of Severely Handicapped Children and Its Meaning for Other Moral Questions** (New York: Paulist Press, 1976); Weber, "Infant Treatment Decisions: Ethics and Cost," **Health Progress** (December 1984), pp. 28–31.

[28]John R. Connery, S.J., "Prolonging Life: The Duty and Its Limits," **Linacre Quarterly** 47 (May 1980), pp. 151–165; Connery, "Prolonging Life: The Duty and Its Limits," in **Moral Responsibility in Prolonging Life Decisions,** eds. Donald G. McCarthy and Albert S. Moraczewski (St. Louis: Pope John

XXIII Center, 1981), pp. 125–138; Connery, "Quality of Life," **Linacre Quarterly** 53 (1986), pp. 26–32. Fr. Connery died on Christmas Eve, 1987.

[29]Donald G. McCarthy, "Treating Defective Newborns: Who Judges Extraordinary Means?" **Hospital Progress** 62 (December 1981), pp. 45–49 + ; Donald G. McCarthy, "Care of Severely Defective Newborn Babies," in **Moral Responsibility in Prolonging Life Decisions,** eds. Donald G. McCarthy and Albert Moraczewski (St. Louis: Pope John XXIII Center, 1981), pp. 213–226.

[30]Reich, "Quality of Life and Defective Newborn Children," p. 499.

[31]Connery, "Prolonging Life," **Linacre Quarterly,** pp. 153–155.

[32]McCarthy, "Care of Severely Defective Newborn Babies," p. 217; Donald McCarthy, "Treating Defective Newborns," pp. 46, 49; similar ideas in Connery, "Prolonging Life," **Linacre Quarterly,** p. 155; Reich and Ost, "Infants: Ethical Perspectives," p. 728; Weber, **Who Shall Live?** pp. 90–91.

[33]Reich and Ost, "Infants: Ethical Perspectives," p. 728.

[34]Ibid.; Weber's definition [**Who Shall Live?** p. 93] is similar: "Excessive burden," indicating extraordinary and optional means, is defined in terms of a "long, drawn-out battle against death or if the treatment itself results in a severe and permanent handicap."

[35]McCarthy, "Introduction to Prolonging Life Issues" and "Theological and Pastoral Dimensions of Prolonging Life Decisions," in **New Technologies of Birth and Death** (St. Louis: Pope John XXIII Center, 1980), pp. 140–143, 178–183.

[36]McCarthy, "Treating Defective Newborns," p. 47;

McCarthy, "Care of Severely Defective Newborn Babies," p. 218.

[37]Reich, "On the Birth," p. 11; Reich, "Testimony," p. 55; Reich, "Quality of Life and Defective Newborn Children," p. 507; cited in Weber, **Who Shall Live?** p. 68; comments about "resiliency" are from McCarthy, "Care of Severely Defective Newborn Babies," pp. 213–214; McCarthy, "Treating Defective Newborns," p. 45.

[38]Connery, "Prolonging Life," **Linacre Quarterly,** p. 159; McCarthy, "Care of Severely Defective Newborn Babies," pp. 215–216; McCarthy, "Treating Defective Newborns," pp. 45–46; Andre E. Hellegers, "What Is 'Extraordinary' in Maintaining Life?" **Ob. Gyn. News** 8 (July 15, 1973), p. 15.

[39]Pius XII, "Prolongation of Life," pp. 395–396.

[40]Reich and Ost, "Infants: Ethical Perspectives," p. 728; Reich, "Quality of Life," pp. 494–495; Reich, "Testimony," p. 57; Weber, **Who Shall Live?** pp. 95, 97–98; Weber, "Infant Treatment Decisions: Ethics and Cost"; McCarthy, "Care of Severely Defective Newborn Babies," p. 224; McCarthy, "Treating Defective Newborns," p. 49; Ashley and O'Rourke, **Health Care Ethics** (1978), p. 389.

[41]Weber, **Who Shall Live?** p. 97.

[42]Reich and Ost, "Infants: Ethical Perspectives," p. 728.

[43]Ashley and O'Rourke, **Health Care Ethics** (1978), p. 389.

[44]Reich, "Quality of Life," p. 506.

[45]McCarthy, "Care of Severely Defective Newborn Babies," p. 218; McCarthy, "Treating Defective Newborns," p. 47; similar to Weber, **Who Shall Live?** pp. 37, 67.

[46]Connery, "Prolonging Life," **Linacre Quarterly,** p. 154.

[47]Connery, "Prolonging Life," in **Moral Responsibility**, p. 134; Connery, "Quality of Life," esp. pp. 31–32.

[48]Weber, **Who Shall Live?** pp. 12, 92; McCarthy, "Care of Severely Defective Newborn Babies," p. 218; Reich and Ost, "Infants: Ethical Perspectives," p. 728.

[49]Germain Grisez and Joseph M. Boyle, Jr., **Life and Death with Liberty and Justice** (Notre Dame: University of Notre Dame Press, 1979), pp. 270–271.

[50]Connery, "Prolonging Life," **Linacre Quarterly**, p. 159; see also Gerald Kelly, "The Duty of Using Artificial Means," pp. 211–212: "In one of Fr. McFadden's discussion problems the doctor expresses the view that it is not necessary to place a monstrosity in a heating bassinet; but Fr. McFadden points out that this is an ordinary means of sustaining infant life and that its use is obligatory even in the case of monstrosities."

[51]Reich, "Life: The Quality of Life," p. 833; Weber, **Who Shall Live?** pp. 45–52.

[52]Quality of Life ethics are critiqued in Reich, "Testimony," pp. 55–58; Guentert and Reich, "Should We Let That Child Die?" pp. 6–13; Reich, "Quality of Life," pp. 490–510; Reich, "Life: The Quality of Life," pp. 829–840; Reich, "Infants: Ethical Perspectives," pp. 728–735; Weber, **Who Shall Live?** pp. 41–52, 65–72, 78–82; McCarthy, "Treating Defective Newborns," pp. 45–46, 49, 54; McCarthy, "Care of Severely Defective Newborn Babies," pp. 215–217, 224–225. Some of the authors mentioned as Quality of Life consequentialists are Richard A. McCormick, Albert Jonsen, Michael Garland, John Lorber, Michael Tooley, Joseph Fletcher, and H. Tristam Engelhardt, Jr. It is my contention that some of these, perhaps all, escape the label "consequentialist" in any pure form (see Chs. 3 and 4).

[53]Ashley and O'Rourke, **Health Care Ethics** (1978), pp. 387–390; rev. ed. (1982), pp. 382–385; See also **Ethics of Health Care** (1986), pp. 201–205.

[54]Bernard Haering, "The Death of Man," in **Medical Ethics** (Notre Dame: Fides Publishers, 1973), pp. 130–151; Bernard Haering, "Bioethics," in **Free & Faithful In Christ** (New York: Crossroad Publishing Co, 1981), III: 4–113, esp. 98–105.

[55]Haering, "Bioethics," p. 102.

[56]Haering, "The Death of Man," p. 141.

[57]Thomas O'Donnell, S.J., "Catholic Thought on Man's Duty to Prolong His Life: An Historical Review," p. 8; O'Donnell, **Medicine and Christian Morality** (1976), pp. 53–55; O'Donnell, "Catholic Historical Perspective," p. 167.

[58]O'Donnell, **Medicine and Christian Morality** (1976), p. 54.

[59]O'Donnell, **The Medical-Moral Newsletter** 11 (October 1974), p. 5.

[60]Congregation for the Doctrine of the Faith, "Vatican Declaration on Euthanasia," **Origins** 10 (August 14, 1980), pp. 154–157, quote from p. 156.

[61]James W. Gaffney, "The Vatican Declaration on Euthanasia and Some Reflections on Christian Ethical Methodology," **Thought** 57 (December 1982), pp. 416–417; Richard A. McCormick, S.J., "Notes on Moral Theology 1980: 'Life and Its Preservation,'" **Theological Studies** 42 (March 1981), pp. 101–102.

[62]Grisez and Boyle, **Life and Death with Liberty and Justice;** Joseph M. Boyle, Jr., "On Killing and Letting Die," **New Scholasticism** (Fall 1977), pp. 433–452; Joseph M. Boyle, Jr.,

"Quality of Life Standards and Withholding Life Saving Treatment," **Proceedings of the American Catholic Philosophical Association** 53 (1979), pp. 150–157; Joseph M. Boyle, Jr., "Treating Defective Newborns: Who Decides? On What Basis?" **Hospital Progress** 63 (August 1982), pp. 34–37, 61; Germain Grisez, "The Value of Life: A Sketch," **Philosophy in Context** 2 (1973), pp. 7–15; Germain Grisez and Russell Shaw, **Beyond the New Morality,** 1st ed. (Notre Dame: University of Notre Dame Press, 1974); Germain Grisez, **The Way of the Lord Jesus, Vol. I: Christian Moral Principles** (Chicago: Franciscan Herald Press, 1983).

[63]Grisez and Boyle, **Life and Death**, pp. 260–261; Boyle, "Quality of Life," p. 154.

[64]Ibid., pp. 268–272.

[65]Boyle, "Quality of Life," pp. 153–154; Boyle, "On Killing and Letting Die," p. 439.

[66]Weber, **Who Shall Live?** pp. 84–85.

[67]Thomas Aquinas, **Summa Theologiae**, Blackfriars Edition (New York: McGraw-Hill Book Co., 1963ff), vol. 38, II, IIae, Question 64, article 7. The following two articles offer the polar parameters for more recent debates concerning the origins and meaning of the principle of Double Effect: J.T. Mangan, "An Historical Analysis of the Principle of Double Effect," **Theological Studies** 10 (1949), pp. 41–61; J. Ghoos, "L'Acte a double effet—Etude de theologie positive," **Ephemerides Theologicae Lovaniensis** 27 (1951), pp. 30–52. The controversy surrounding the validity of the double effect principle is ongoing. The following sources are beneficial anthologies of the controversy: Charles E. Curran and Richard A. McCormick, eds., **Readings in Moral Theology, No. 1: Moral Norms and Catholic Tradition** (New York: Paulist Press, 1979); Richard A.

McCormick and Paul Ramsey, eds., **Doing Evil to Achieve Good** (Chicago: Loyola University Press, 1978); Charles E. Curran, ed., **Absolutes in Moral Theology?** (Westport, Conn.: Greenwood Press, 1968).

[68]Leo XIII **Rerum Novarum** (1891); Pius XI, **Quadragesimo Anno** (1931) and **Divini Redemptoris** (1937); John XXIII, **Mater et Magistra** (1961) and **Pacem in Terris** (1963); Vatican II, **Gaudium et Spes** (1965); Paul VI, **Populorum Progressio** (1967) and **Octagesimo Adveniens** (1971); Synod of Bishops, **Justice in the World** (1971); John Paul II, **Redemptor Hominis** (1979) and **Laborem Exercens** (1981).

[69]Ramsey, **Ethics at the Edges of Life**, p. 153.

[70]President's Commission, **Deciding to Forego**, pp. 60–62, 82–89; Beauchamp and Childress, **Principles of Biomedical Ethics**, p. 117; Congregation for the Doctrine of the Faith, "Vatican Declaration on Euthanasia," p. 156; Reich and Ost, "Infants: Ethical Perspectives," p. 729. Reich and Ost paraphrase their critics with the "surrounded by ambiguities" phrase; "Ordinary and Extraordinary Means—Editorial," **Journal of Medical Ethics** 7 (June 1981), p. 56; Edward W. Keyserlingk, **Sanctity of Life or Quality of Life in the Context of Ethics, Medicine, and Law** (Ottawa: Law Reform Commission of Canada, 1979), p. 131.

[71]Ramscy, **The Patient as Person**, pp. 121–123; Veatch, **Death, Dying, and the Biological Revolution**, p. 106; President's Commission, **Deciding to Forego**, pp. 84–85.

[72]Gerald Kelly, "The Duty of Using Artificial Means," esp. pp. 204–206.

[73]E. Genicot and J. Salsmans, **Institutiones Theologiae Moralis** (Bruxelles: L'Edition Universelle, 17th ed., 1951), I: p.

364; H. Jone and U. Adelman, **Moral Theology** (Westminster, Md.: Newman Press, 1948), p. 210.

[74]Connery, "Prolonging Life," **Linacre Quarterly**, pp. 155–156.

[75]Reich, "On the Birth," p. 10; Warren T. Reich, "Dignity in Death and Life," **New York Times** (16 January 1973), Op. Ed. page.

[76]O'Donnell, "Catholic Thought on Man's Duty," p. 8; O'Donnell, "A Catholic Historical Perspective," p. 168.

[77]O'Donnell, **The Medical-Moral Newsletter** 11 (October 1974), p. 6.

[78]Ramsey, "Prolonged Dying: Not Medically Indicated," p. 14.

[79]Atkinson, "Theological History of Catholic Teaching on Prolonging Life," esp. pp. 105–110.

[80]Connery, "Prolonging Life," in **Moral Responsibility**, pp. 132–133: "I think a proxy could be justifiably influenced in his decision by a patient's handicap if it would make the use of the means considerably more difficult, or even more so, if it made their use ineffective. . . . The recent Spring case is a good example of how a handicap can add to the burden of treatment. The inability of the patient, because of his senility, to understand what was going on made the hemodialysis treatment very trying, even resulting in violent reactions on his part. It is understandable that a proxy might not give consent to treatment in these circumstances even though the ordinary patient would generally consent to it." (p. 132).

[81]Gerald Kelly, "The Duty of Using Artificial Means," pp. 216–220. Gerald Kelly admitted that mandating insulin for a di-

abetic patient with terminal cancer is somehow inordinate and perhaps ought to be optional.

82Andre E. Hellegers, "What Is 'Extraordinary' in Maintaining Life?" **Ob. Gyn. News** 8 (July 15, 1973), pp. 14–15; Andre E. Hellegers, "The Johns Hopkins Case," **Ob. Gyn. News** 8 (June 15, 1973), pp. 40–41.

83Ibid., p. 15.

84Reich, "Quality of Life," p. 508; Paul Ramsey questions the consistency of this third category with the above stated restriction that the measurement of qualitative burden must be directly related to the means itself. Ramsey suggests that Reich needs to further clarify this category lest he be adopting Richard McCormick's relational potential standard, not restricted to means. [Ramsey, **Ethics at the Edges of Life,** p. 181.]

85"Ordinary and Extraordinary Means—Editorial," p. 56.

Chapter Three

Projected Quality of the Patient's Life
(Not Restricted to Means Causation)

"There is no such thing as a life not worth living." "Every life is worthwhile." "All life is meaningful." These are some of the standard "slogans" or arguments set forth by impassioned critics against all efforts to consciously incorporate quality of life factors into the treatment/nontreatment equation. The core question that must be asked in response is: "Worthwhile and meaningful **to whom?**" If one means: Is life qua life, as an abstraction within the created or natural order, always meaningful or a worthwhile value on some theoretical scale of realities to be esteemed? One may rightly answer "yes." However, if we enflesh that abstract life principle in particular, historically and circumstantially contexted human beings, then one might well ask: Is that basic or biological "life" always meaningful and worthwhile **to and for this given patient?** For example, does biosfunctioning, sustained only by the lower brain stem, have "meaning" or "worth" to a patient whose upper brain is totally extinguished and who lives with "a permanent loss of consciousness"? Or if someone is suffering excruciating and irremediable pain, does continued life, in terms of heart and lung pumping, have meaning or value to that patient? Or simply in the case of imminently dying patients, is it conceivable that for some the meaning or worth of prolonged life in terms of basic vital signs is of far "less" value to them than if their earthly future offered more promise?

Such logical contextualizing of the meaning and value of "life" in the biological sense within the framework of one's "life" in the historical and holistic sense is at the core of the "projected quality of the patient's life" criteria to be presented here. While "life" as vital signs is always a value to be esteemed in a theoretical sense, at times it is ethically appropriate to sacrifice it or at least to choose other values before it for the sake of one's total well-being. The same patient-centered burden-to-benefit calculus advocated by Reich, Weber, Connery, and McCarthy is carried over by "projected quality of the patient's life" proponents like McCormick, Paris, Jonsen, Garland, Shaw, Duff, Campbell, and Lorber, though now minus the "caused by means" restriction.

What emerges is a treatment/nontreatment standard rooted in the inherent value of all human life, an essential belief in the principle of Totality, and a scrupulous effort to discern what amalgam of handicaps and extraordinary burden are necessary to decide that further efforts to prolong the physiological aspects of life are not in the patient's best interest. In short, when, if ever, is the quality of one's life so inordinately wretched **for the patient**, regardless of potential medical benefit and regardless of whether the means cause or merely perpetuate such burden, that death or at least a shorter life span is to be welcomed, not forestalled? If such inhumane kinds or qualities of life can be defined, should not that patient or one's advocate be empowered to accept/forego further life-sustaining efforts accordingly?

The "projected quality of a patient's life" approach is grounded in four fundamental presuppositions. This chapter will open with a brief presentation of those four underlying values, which, to a large extent, reflect the core presuppositions of the previous chapter. In the second section a series of authors will be presented representing the spectrum of opinion as to what neonatal cases constitute lives qualitatively extraordinary and overburdened. While Varga, McCormick, Paris, Arras, Hellegers, Keyserlingk, and Veatch champion a stricter definition of a quality of life exempting one from the obligation to treat, Shaw, Duff, Campbell, Lorber, and Weir represent the broader end of the spectrum. The final critique section will be two-pronged—a critique of the "projected quality of the patient's life" approach in general, as well as of the so-called restrictive versus broader interpretations of what constitutes an excessively burdened quality of life.

Fundamental Principles, Presuppositions, or Values

The "projected quality of the patient's life" standard to be surveyed here rests on four fundamental presuppositions:

1. the inherent value of every embodied human life, with a **prima facie** mandate to sustain and prolong life accordingly;

2. the Principle of Totality, whereby one's organs and bodily life are subservient to the total well-being of the person as a multidimensional (physiological, psychological, social, and spiritual) whole;

3. a primary, quasi-exclusive focus on the patient's best interest in biomedical decision making (the only exception being those cases in which the finitude of societal resources necessitates limitations on a patient's access to any and all treatment);

4. a commitment to alleviating human pain and suffering within the context of fostering one's holistic well-being.

A contemporary proponent of the ordinary/extraordinary means distinction would likewise adopt all four. For that matter, the first three received extensive treatment in the opening section of the previous chapter, necessitating only brief summarization in what follows. The fourth, a commitment to alleviating pain and suffering, can rightly be ascribed to all four treatment standards surveyed in this volume. However, it is cited here as a fundamental value for "projected quality of the patient's life" proponents because of its primary significance in cases in which one's condition itself is considered inordinately painful or suffering-laden and thus the basis for nontreatment.

1. Quality of life proponents Albert Jonsen and Michael Garland assert that every infant "requires by its very existence to be approached with attitudes of respect, consideration, and care."[1] The infant is designated as a person, a rights-bearing being, regardless of functional ability or social utility. This inherent value or dignity is the core principle which undergirds all patient-centered quality of life ethics. However, as noted earlier, "life" is an ambiguous concept. In an abstract sense life in itself is a powerful force commanding unmitigated respect. For religious believers "life" is grace incarnate, the spirit or breath of God, and as such is holy and merits reverence. Philosophically, "life" is that mysterious force which animates sentient beings and makes them "more" or "higher" than lifeless objects.

But respect for the inherent dignity of **human** life implies historical context and particularity. Once life is incarnated in specific human beings it becomes a value in context. As Richard McCormick sees it, "life is indeed a basic and a precious good, but a good to be preserved precisely as the condition of other values."[2] The Christian tradition, according to McCormick, sees biological life as a fundamental value, but not an absolute one.[3] Nor is physical death the ultimate evil. At times, physical and/or mental afflictions may be so burdensome to a given patient that death might be desirable, viewed as a benefit, or at least as the lesser evil—hence, the old adage "a blessing in disguise." Therefore, the quality of life proponents to be surveyed in this chapter subscribe to the obligation to sustain and prolong the physiological aspect of "life" as a **prima facie,** not an absolute duty.

Georgetown Jesuit Walter Burghardt, in a somewhat homiletic treatment of the subject, differentiates three valid and valuable aspects of the good called "life"—sheer life, good life, and eternal life.[4] Quality of life proponents prioritize these meanings or aspects of life in ascending order. At times sheer life (vital signs) may be sacrificed [at least indirectly] for or superseded by good life (one's earthly human flourishing). For believers even that is subservient to one's prospects for eternal life (salvation/life's highest goal). According to quality of life proponents this is not a negation of "life," but an **ordo bonorum** (better ordering) in which "sheer life" is the least though not insignificant element in the progressive movement from mere existence to full human flourishing and eternal salvation.[5] In short, a quality of life approach to nontreatment questions need not deny the inherent value of the individual in asking whether continued embodied existence will offer such a valuable individual "any hope of sharing those values for which physical life is the fundamental condition."[6]

2. The inherent value and dignity of every human being is the presumed starting point to be balanced off with and, at times, against that individual's holistic and eternal well-being. Thus the principle of Totality, which is a cornerstone for the ordinary/extraordinary means tradition, serves a similar balancing function here. As noted in Chapter Two, Pius XII asserted that "before all else" one

> should consider the whole man, in the unity of his person, that is to say, not merely in his physical condition but his psychological state as well as his spiritual and moral ideals and his place in society.[7]

In other places he spoke of one's organism being subordinate to "the spiritual end(s) of the person."[8] "Projected quality of the patient's life" proponents rely heavily on this broader interpretation of the principle of Totality to justify decisions to cease or forego potentially life-sustaining treatments. The presupposition in favor of life prolongation yields to a patient-oriented burden/benefit calculus in those instances when the quality or condition of one's "life" gravely inhibits or overburdens one's human flourishing and/or progress toward the kingdom.

3. In its 1983 study **Deciding to Forego Life-Sustaining Treatment** the President's Commission asserted that for all competent patients two values ought to guide decision making—"promoting patient welfare" and "respecting patient self-determination."[9] While the latter might be interpreted as approbation for absolute patient autonomy, in context the Commission carefully hems in a competent patient's liberty with determination of competency and counter-balancing rights/duties of the health care system and society. The Hippocratic tradition's non-maleficence bottom line inhibits granting full freedom to questionably competent patients or to obviously self-destructive decisions. So while a patient's right to participate in decisions about one's own future ought generally to be respected (principle of informed consent), ultimately "promoting patient welfare" dominates this balance with "patient self-determination."

In the case of non-competent patients, the Commission recognizes two standards that roughly parallel the above values—"best interests" and "substituted judgment." In those cases in which a now non-competent patient was formerly competent, family or court-appointed guardians ought to act as one's substitute, granting or withholding permissions for treatment based on that patient's previously expressed desires, values, and stated intentions. However, in the cases in which no prior wishes exist, particularly the cases of handicapped infants and others who have never been competent, the Commission recommends that parents or guardians "make a choice for the patient that seeks to implement what is in that person's best interests." Such decisions ought to rest on "objective, societally shared criteria," not on the autonomy or self-determination principle.[10] On certain points no societal consensus may exist. Lest patients in such "gray" areas be sustained coercively beyond a point at which many competent patients would say "halt," parents in consultation with physicians and possibly overseen by court review should be allowed some prudential leeway for interpreting a patient's best interest in context.

The "patient's best interest" is the primary, quasi-absolute focus of decision making for all the scholars to be surveyed in this chapter. The title "projected quality **of the patient's life**" for this third type is more cumbersome than simply saying "quality of life," but the emphasis on **the patient's life** is fundamental to good medical practice and to the ethics of all grouped under this banner.[11] By focusing on the patient's best interest, particularly in the case of children, this standard avoids the slippery slope to justifications based on the well-being of other interested parties—parents, fellow siblings, or society at large—over against the patient's needs and interests. While some proponents of the quality of life standard to be surveyed here allow social factors to be incorporated, these are limited to those social burdens impinging directly on the non-competent patient's best interests, viewed holistically.

4. The fourth value underlying the "projected quality of the patient's life" position is a direct outgrowth of the formal principles of beneficence and non-maleficence. It is the presumed duty of guardians and medical personnel not only to save and prolong life, not only to effect maximum health potential, but also to comfort, console, and **alleviate suffering** as much as is humanly possible. As John Arras phrases it, "We continue to believe that pain and suffering are evil, and that beneficence largely consists in abolishing, or at least ameliorating, these twin

scourges of humankind."[12] This core value is certainly not unique to the "projected quality of the patient's life" standard, but it does serve in a unique way to ground its assertion that certain kinds or qualities of life, irrespective of means causation, may already be extraordinarily burdened by pain or psychological suffering. If some kinds of physical or psychic suffering are in fact irremediable (a debated "if"), and if the efforts to prolong life serve only to perpetuate a life plagued by such suffering, then is it not morally permissible, even obligatory, to cease treatment, indirectly shortening "life" as bios, in the name of "Life" as one's totality or holistic best interests?

Christians have traditionally seen human suffering as potentially positive, redemptive, linked to the salvific suffering of Christ.[13] As one commentator notes, "the turf of suffering provides virtue's breeding ground."[14] Nevertheless, it would be incorrect to read into this that physical pain or psychic suffering is somehow intrinsically good or categorically to be valued. Eschewing as sado-masochistic a philosophy or piety that imbues pain and suffering with value in itself, "projected quality of the patient's life" proponents see pain and suffering as basic disvalues or evils to be alleviated if at all possible.

Unavoidable suffering may be accepted or endured by some competent patients with creative determination, thus deepening or molding their human spirits. However, such saintly forbearance in no way elevates the precipitating pain or suffering to the status of a good in itself or even of neutrality. Irritated nerve endings or tormented psyches contribute only indirectly to human well-being, and then only if the sufferer is so graced as to be able to impute meaning into one's ill fortune. For every "Helen Keller" there may also be equally plagued individuals lacking the strength of character to deal creatively with insurmountable pain or extraordinary suffering. Mainline Christianity has consistently upheld "the Christian and human prudence" reflected in the societal use of pain-killing medications to alleviate or suppress the suffering related to disease.

With regard to non-competents, especially babies, "one can reasonably presume that they wish to take these painkillers. . . ."[15] Why? Infants at best are "conscious" in the generic sense of being cognizant of sensory input, but they are "pre-conscious" or "non-conscious" in terms of conceptualization and intentionality. From the perspective of these patients, pain and suffering can serve no positive purpose. For them, as for their severely retarded fellow non-competents, pain and suffering are to be alleviated or minimized as much as possible within the limits of their holistic best interests.

Before concluding this brief treatment of pain and suffering, it is important to note that "pain" in terms of throbbing nerve endings is not the totality of what constitutes unbearable human suffering.[16] Marquette ethicist Daniel Maguire cites Huntington's disease as an illustration of a minimally painful illness fraught with "unique suffering." He points out that the disease involves a series of uniquely dehumanizing burdens—continuous, involuntary and uncoordinated movements of the limbs and face, loss of articulation, and marked tendencies to moodiness, irascibility, and disorientation. He concludes that "the final phase of this disease merits the term macabre."[17] It is conceivable that a competent, life-respecting patient would find such involuntary movement and moods to be "extraordinarily" burdensome, painful in the broader sense of human suffering. While it is difficult to decipher what sort of mental anguish, if any, goes on in the mind of a newborn who is constantly poked with tubes, kept away from the home environment, and subjected to endless series of tests, one might argue that such treatment, even if not physically painful, is experienced as "abuse" rather than affectionate "care."[18] In short, "pain-management," however pharmaceutically, surgically, and psychologically perfected, is not identical with "suffering-management."

The proponents of a "projected quality of the patient's life" standard are thus closely related in fundamental presuppositions to the scholars surveyed under the contemporary ordinary/extraordinary means banner. Both ride a middle course in respecting the inherent dignity or personhood of every living human being, while at the same time seeing that person's rightful interest in treatment as hinging on a holistic or totality-based interpretation of his/her wider best interests. Excruciating pain or irremediable suffering calls for palliative relief, even at the risk of shortening or perhaps suppressing "sheer life." The direct/indirect distinction, however, is not as paramount as it was for contemporary ordinary/extraordinary means proponents, nor is the "means restriction" essential to judge one's prognosis hopeless or extraordinarily burdened.

Content of a Quality of Life Standard: A Spectrum with Reference to Handicapped Newborns

Numerous prominent physicians and ethicists subscribe somewhat generically to quality of life standards. Some, like Drs. Gordon Avery, Clement Smith, and Judson Randolph, adopt phrases like "meaningful life" and a "life worth living," without unpacking their content.[19] Drs. Norman Fost and David Roy each speak broadly of extensive handicapped conditions which would in themselves make further life fall far short of the purposes to which biological human life is ordained.[20] Nor are these responses atypical.

In the spring of 1975 a nationwide survey was conducted of the "attitudes and practices" of American pediatric surgeons and pediatric chiefs of staff in reference to nontreatment decisions for handicapped infants,[21] and 83% of the surgeons and 81% of the pediatricians answered "no" to the question, "Do you believe that the life of each and every newborn infant should be saved if it is within our ability to do so?" In a related question which asked them to prioritize a list of criteria justifying allowing "certain severely damaged infants to die by withholding treatment," 83.6% of the pediatricians and 90.7% of the surgeons gave primacy to "potential quality of life." "Probable I.Q." and "possible adverse effects on the family" vied for second place. Other similar, regional surveys bear out the general accuracy of these statistics for the American pediatric medical community.[22] In short, some form of the quality of life standard, even when intuited or only semi-reflectively analyzed, seems to be the dominant criteria standard operative in American pediatric practice.

That is perhaps one reason why the President's Commission adopted a patient-centered quality of life approach in regard to handicapped newborns in their official report, **Deciding to Forego Life-Sustaining Treatment.** Cognizant of the fact that many life-saving therapies will leave a child with permanent handicaps, either related to the therapy **or from the underlying defect itself,** the Commission noted that "one of the most troubling and persistent issues" is whether and to what extent one's handicaps should be considered in deciding to accept or forego treatment. The Commission, in a tacit quality of life statement, concludes restrictively that "such permanent handicaps justify a decision not to provide life-sustaining treatment only when they are so severe that continued existence would not be a net benefit for the infant."[23] Admitting that such a guideline is "inevitably somewhat subjective and imprecise in actual application," the Commission chose a generic mid-course between forced treatment for all and accepting any reason for nontreatment as valid by way of some libertarian concept of parental autonomy.

Mindful of the patient's best interest, viewed from a "totality" perspective, what quality of life or amalgam of qualities is essential to make life even minimally 'meaningful' or 'valuable' **to the patient?** A two-tiered analysis seems inevitable. First, are there any human, physiologically-rooted functions or faculties, beyond 'sheer life' itself, that are required for even minimal participation in life's uniquely human values? Second, even if a patient possesses at least this minimal ability to participate in the goods of human flourishing, what configuration of bodily impairments, pain, and 'cost' would be necessary to override or neutralize one's further interest in vital signs prolongation? The latter question is identical to the determination of excessive burden in the ordinary/extraordinary means tradition. Regardless of a patient's potential for biological life, when, if ever, are burdens so excessive that one's best interest is being subordinated or even negated by the mere effort to survive and/or to cope? Rather than neatly spacing themselves across a spectrum, the scholars to be surveyed here gravitate toward two poles, both patient-centered.

1. A Restrictive Approach

At the more restrictive or conservative pole of the "projected quality of the patient's life" spectrum are a number of ethicists and scholars who define "meaningful life" or a life which generally mandates treatment in terms of some minimal capacity for human "consciousness" or relationality or both. These scholars attempt to clarify which physiologically-based functions are essential to declare a human infant more than "living" vital signs, more than brain-stem sustained reflexive processes, more than a person solely in an essential or inherent sense. None of these scholars, however, denies basic humanity or personhood to an infant lacking this minimal consciousness or relational potential. They merely propose that such an infant ceases to have a compelling personal reason for interminable life prolongation by medical means. Any treatment is categorically burdensome/too costly for relatively no benefit.

Fordham philosopher Andrew C. Varga suggests that the purpose of medical intervention in the case of handicapped newborns "is not just the assurance of vegetative survival but also the assurance of at least some degree of rational and interrelational development."[24] While former Kennedy Center colleagues James Childress and Tom Beauchamp are reluctant to adopt the "quality of life" label, they too uphold the position that further treatment may offer no appreciable benefit **to the patient** if "there is a justifiable prediction of irreversible loss of mentation."[25] If there is "no reasonable prospect of recovery of cognitive, sapient life," then further life-sustaining efforts may be judged non-obligatory. In the concluding section of a lengthy study done for the Law Reform Commission of Canada, Edward Keyserlingk similarly declares that "a minimal potential capacity **to experience and to relate**" ought to hold "the determinative place" in deciding whether treatment is in the infant's best interest or not. According to Keyserlingk, "both human experience and religious belief have long and indisputably argued that the meaning and purpose of life is found in relating with others (religion would add, with God, as well)."[26] Jesuit moral theologian Richard McCormick would heartily concur.

In July 1974 McCormick published a controversial five page article, "To Save or Let Die," simultaneously in **America** and the **Journal of the American Medical Association**.[27] In this brief treatise, and in at least twenty subsequent articles, McCormick sets forth "broad guidelines" for a quality of life ethic of treatment/nontreatment in reference to handicapped newborns.[28] McCormick distinguishes between two sets of human capacities or conditions: those which allow us to do things well, easily, comfortably, and efficiently, and those which allow us to do them **at all**.[29] He perceives contemporary life or death medical decisions involving "quality" as pertaining primarily to the second set. While optimum development of one's physiological and mental capabilities is a valid goal for medicine to foster, human life has "meaning" to the patient, albeit limited, at the level of the minimal ability to consciously participate at all. McCormick believes that even stripped of all idyllic aspirations, the core "meaning, substance, and consummation of life is found in human **relationships,** and the qualities of justice, respect, concern, compassion, and support that surround them."[30]

In an all too brief and somewhat sketchy treatment of the Scriptures, the speeches of Pius XII, and the theology of Karl Rahner, McCormick asserts that this emphasis on relationality, particularly that human relationship called "love," sums up succinctly the substance and goal of human life from a Judaeo-Christian perspective.[31] Scripturally, he draws this from Jesus' own ethical synthesis when asked: "What is the greatest of all the commandments?" Jesus brought together for the first time the **Shema** command to love God wholeheartedly (Dt 6:4–5) with the priestly command "to love your neighbor as yourself" (Lev 19:18).[32] If the essential relationship of **love** (for others, for God, as for self) is the benchmark of a Christian life lived humanly and spiritually well, then McCormick concludes that a life lacking the basic capacity for such responsive love is a human life with no earthly potential, no personal future **for the patient,** except death and whatever awaits thereafter.

In this temporal, embodied, historical world, McCormick proposes that one's ability to love God is inextricably linked to human relationships, one's ability to love the neighbor. He quotes from the First Epistle of John as a proof-text for this linkage:

> If any man says "I love God" and hates his brother, he is a liar. For he who loves not his brother, whom he sees, how can he love God whom he does not see? (1 Jn 4:20–21).

The measure with which we love our fellow human beings is the embodiment and reflection of our love response to the invisible God. Attributing this insight to Karl Rahner, McCormick concludes that when this potentiality is totally absent or would be totally subordinated to the mere effort for survival because of the [burdened/pained] condition of the individual, that life can be said "to have achieved its potential."

To have achieved one's potential, or, in some sense, to be without further embodied relational potential, is not to say one's "life" is meaningless in a theoretical or ontic sense. However, the fundamental inability to experientially "relate with one's environment," even in a minimal, sensory way, would, for McCormick, indicate a life of little or no further value **to the patient** so mentally deprived. The best treatment for the patient would seem to be nontreatment, even though interim therapies or life-sustaining equipment could probably prolong such a life indefinitely.

Fellow Jesuit and sometimes collaborator John J. Paris also asserts that "love," enfleshed in justice, gratitude, forebearance, and charity, is the chief role and purpose of human activity. To be fundamentally incapable of active participation in love relationships is to have no **subjective** role or interest in prolonged earthly living. Paris finds theological grounding for this assertion in the stewardship and journey metaphors. Life is both a gift from God entrusted to us as well as a journey of indeterminate length "back to God." In this interim between creation and the end of time we are responsible for caring for our own bodies and holistic well-being. Noting Teilhard de Chardin's admonition against too easily caving in, in the face of illness, as if God wills our premature demise, Paris proposes that "our task in the face of the forces of diminishment is to struggle with all our energy, talents, and might to reverse it."[33]

If, however, one has exhausted these, or worse yet has lost the very capacity to consciously participate in "the good fight," it is permissible to cease further fruitless efforts for such a patient, accepting the inevitable as part of the Divine plan. Citing **The Divine Milieu** as his source, Paris suggests that there comes a point in everyone's life, including "the one day old infant whose potential for future relationships, for loving, and for being loved does not exist or is submerged in the mere struggle to survive," when the journey has reached its end.[34] These diminished lives do not cease to have inherent value precisely because they are acts or creations of Divine love. They do, however, cease to have any potential or human value for the embodied patient and, therefore, in the patient's best interest the best treatment is non-treatment. It is Paris' belief that the potential benefit derivable from life-saving treatment is in proportion to one's capacity to consciously enter into human relationships. If that potential is non-existent, extinguished, or overcome by pain and burden, then God's ultimate will for the patient is best served by non-treatment. "In fact, to treat is to do a disservice to the humanity of the individual involved."[35]

In the introductory chapter of **Human Medicine,** Protestant ethicist James B. Nelson similarly asserts that in Christian ethics "we are concerned not only about human physical existence but also about that quality of existence in which the individual has some meaningful consciousness, self-awareness, and capacity for interpersonal relationship and communication."[36] He suggests that in the seriously and permanently brain-injured patient, "personal existence is gone both in actuality and potentiality." To be personally human is to be **social.** We are humanized, brought into being as fully human, "only in a web of personal relationships." Called by God, aware of self and of others around us, we are created in and for community. If social existence is indeed fundamental, then medical decisions ought to respect and nurture that possibility. A patient's wholeness ought never be confused with one's "compound of chemicals" (physicality). Nelson agrees with Paris that to do so "dehumanizes" that patient.

All of these religiously-grounded rationales for seeing "relationality" [measured by some minimal level of "consciousness" or brain activity] as the core meaning of embodied existence lead directly back to the principle of Totality discussed earlier. The total good to which body parts and functioning itself are subordinate is that of the whole person, one's best interests holistically considered.[37] According to Martin Nolan's treatment of the topic, the total good of the whole person "is achieved in actuating oneself in one's innermost reality which is relationship to God and to others." Or again, "the innermost core of all creaturehood is utter relationship."[38] Therefore, as Varga, Keyserlingk, Childress, Beauchamp, McCormick, Paris, and Nelson noted, if one is fundamentally, physiologically incapable of further embodied awareness, response, and communication, however minimally, then one ceases to have a personal interest in prolonged embodiment. Relational communication with God, if still continuing, is transbiological, not essentially dependent on sustained vital signs. Sustained "life" with no potential for embodied relational experience is at best "meaningless" to the patient and at worst a dehumanizing prolongation of "mere life," which has ceased to be of significance for the patient's total or wider well-being.[39] Further treatment becomes relatively nonbeneficial in light of the patient's permanent inability to participate in the activities related to human flourishing.

In "A Proposal for 'Quality of Life' Criteria for Sustaining Life" McCormick claims a practical affinity with Paul Ramsey's two curious exceptions to treatment surveyed earlier—(1) total inability to receive and respond to care and (2) excruciating or intractable pain. If treatment serves only to prolong "a life that is totally without any potential for human experience or relating" or a life of "excruciating, and, therefore, isolating [relation-less] pain," then such treatment would be **nocere** or harm to the patient's best interest, a perversion of good medical practice. "If, however, the life saved will be one without excruciating pain and with some minimal capacity for experience, then one may not conclude that that life has achieved its potential."[40] Unlike Ramsey, McCormick categorically rejects the option of active infanticide. Holding to the direct/indirect distinction between "directly intended killing" and "allowing to die," McCormick upholds foregoing or ceasing treatment in these two instances to allow death to come more quickly, but refuses to condone active killing of the newborn, even under the banner of "the caring thing to do."

In the concluding paragraphs of "To Save or Let Die" McCormick posits several caveats to this **relational potential** criterion or guideline. First, he notes that this guideline is not a detailed rule that exempts one from prudential judgments concerning which infants are in fact totally unaware and wholly nonrelational. Second, given the fact that an infant has no past to build on, no known aspirations out of which to weave his/her own interpretation of benefit or best interest, decisions made for him/her cannot be individualized or particularized beyond criteria generalizable to all infants. As a consequence, McCormick asserts that the criteria used to determine minimal capacity to relate "must be the strictest possible" to forestall abuse or well intentioned misprognoses. He concludes that "the very minimum potential for human experiencing or relationship must be seen as sufficient warrant for attempting to save." It is better to err on the side of life-prolongation in borderline cases.[41]

In "To Save or Let Die" McCormick's application of this standard to neonatal cases is disappointing in its brevity (four sentences) and only minimally helpful in deciding what cases might constitute excruciating pain or excessive burden. He leaves to physicians the task of providing "more concrete categories or presumptive biological symptoms" to enflesh what constitutes a totally non-relational and/or an intractably pained mental state.[42] McCormick does plot two extreme cases on the spectrum, without filling in the conflictual middle. At the one extreme is the anencephalic infant, whose lack of neocortical function obviously indicates a life wholly without relational potential. Life-sustaining treatments are therefore optional, even contra-indicated. At the opposite extreme of the handicap spectrum is a "mongoloid" infant or Down's Syndrome child. While retarded mental capacities inhibit these Trisomy 21 victims from higher education and advanced academic achievements, these infants are still "aware," "conscious," and capable of interrelating with their environment and with others. If anything, their capacity for uninhibited "love" is enhanced by the limitation of mental complexity and nuance. Thus, Down's Syndrome alone constitutes neither a life lacking relational potential nor a life excessively burdened by pain or inordinate inconvenience.

In a more recent article, co-authored with John Paris, McCormick categorically excludes omitting life-sustaining interventions "simply because the baby is retarded."[43] Retardation (with a mental capacity somewhere above the anencephalic level) in itself is not an indication for nontreatment. However, retardation may, in some unnamed cases, be one factor in an amalgam of deformities and handicaps that could constitute a life excessively burdened.

In terms of newborn life that is at least minimally relational, McCormick does not delineate which cases, if any, constitute intractably pained existence. Whether he would agree with Ramsey's suggestions of Lesch-Nyhan syndrome or epidermolysis bulloso becomes a matter for conjecture. McCormick and Paris assert that the necessity of repeated cardiac surgery, of low prognosis transplants, of increasingly traumatic oxygenation for low-birthweight babies, or of interminable artificial feeding is a burden which might be labeled "excessive," especially if the expected life can be had only for a relatively brief time.[44] Some cases of necrotizing enterocolitis are illustrative of the artificial feeding for minimal life extension scenario. Beyond this McCormick does not elaborate in detail on neonatal case applications.

Chicago moralist John Dedek, British pediatric surgeon R.B. Zachary, and Louvain graduate Edward J. Mahoney all subscribe to McCormick's relational potential criterion.[45] Likewise,

Dr. Andre Hellegers applauded McCormick's "To Save or Let Die" schema as a "major contribution" to the debate and agreed that in theory an infant's total inability to relate could justify non-treatment. However, Hellegers was quick to add a caveat concerning the medical difficulty and potential abuse of establishing "biological criteria like signs, symptoms, I.Q.s or lab results" to correspond with McCormick's religiously-rooted criterion.[46] Hellegers' core question "How do you, in a newborn, determine the future ability to relate to other humans?" remains a "sticking point" for translating McCormick's theory into medical practice.

In two separate articles philosopher Paul R. Johnson adopts McCormick's **relational potential** criterion and attempts to do just that, to refine and apply it to further specific cases.[47] Johnson hones in on "mental functioning" of the brain as the biological zone for determining an infant's capacity to relate. He rejects other physical deformities or dysfunctions, however lamentable, as irrelevant to the determination of one's minimum relational ability. Using mental retardation as the measure of mental capacities is itself a variable criterion. Given the fact that the range of possible retardation is wide and that the ability of the mentally impaired person "to experience and enjoy human relationships apparently reaches well down the I.Q. scale," Johnson, paralleling the more recent McCormick-Paris article, rejects the generic presence of "mental retardation" as a synonym for "lack of relational potential." He goes on to side with more conservative special educators who believe that infants with low I.Q.s in the 20–35 range are still trainable and ought not, on the basis of I.Q. alone, be labeled "severely or profoundly retarded," particularly if such categories imply no educational therapy. Since "trainable" implies some measure of **relationship** with a human tutor, Johnson concludes that the vast majority of Down's Syndrome babies (I.Q.s usually between 40–60) do have relational potential and that McCormick's lack of relational potential category is not operative until somewhere below 25–30 on a standard I.Q. scale.[48]

Children born with myelomeningocele are admittedly more problematic. At one extreme are those few patients for whom surgery would be useless either because death is imminent or because the lesion and meningocele are so large. At the opposite extreme, some spina bifida lesions are minor, easy to close, and prognosis for a relatively "normal" life is good. In between, as the Lorber-Zachary debate indicates, are a number of infants whose prognoses are debatable. Given shunt treatment for hydrocephalus, few if any would be so mentally retarded as to be non-sapient or wholly unrelatable. However, it is arguable that in addition to spinal deformity, the combination of repeated orthopedic surgery, long hospitalizations, possible paraplegia, repeated shunt replacement for hydrocephalus, possible mental retardation, the inconvenience and embarrassment of incontinence, and the cost of long-term care to oneself or one's loved ones reasonably could be judged by some as excessive burden. Regardless of potential biological benefit (lesion closure), even contemporary ordinary/extraordinary means advocates would concur that the long term prognosis and care for some spina bifida patients with myelomeningocele could perhaps rightly be judged extraordinary in burden over benefit evaluation.

Johnson concludes that except in cases involving anencephaly, exencephaly, or severe collateral physical brain damage, the criterion "total lack of relational potential" is seldom met. The second criterion, "determination of excessive burden and/ or intractable pain," though more common, is "not nearly so prevalent as critics fear would be allowed by McCormick's position."[49]

Beauchamp and Childress suggest that some infants who suffer either Tay-Sachs disease or Lesch-Nyhan syndrome may be judged extraordinarily pained, or so burdened by the condition itself. The former is a disease which involves increasing spasticity and dementia, which usually results in death by the age of three or four. The latter, as cited by Ramsey, is marked by uncontrollable spasms, mental retardation, compulsive self-mutilation, and early death.[50] It is conceivable that in these cases, particularly in the latter stages, the sheer effort to stay alive, coping with pain or suffering, would subvert or even negate any remaining potential to relate and respond to care.

The writings of Kennedy Center scholar Robert Veatch echo the above case applications, though it has been debated whether he ought to be labeled a "projected quality of the patient's life" proponent or an advocate of the ordinary/extraordinary means tradition, complete with the means-related proviso. Specifically with reference to handicapped newborns Veatch speaks of a guardian's right to refuse even life-saving treatments for the infant if it [the treatment] "is unreasonable—because of its uselessness or the burden it generates."[51] However, earlier in the same chapter, as he unpacked the meaning of burden post-treatment, this cause/effect relationship of means to burden is tenuous or even severed. In a subsequent article following the Bloomington "Infant Doe" Case Veatch seems to adopt more openly the quality of the patient's life perspective, irrespective of means causation. In response to the question "What, finally, if the underlying condition itself makes life gravely burdensome even though the treatment proposed itself may be quite simple and painless?" Veatch asserts that while treatment should not be withheld solely because an infant is handicapped, one's handicap ought not be excluded from the amalgam of factors involved in determining whether treatment will or will not be in that patient's holistic best interest.[52]

In May 1974, at Sonoma, California, an interdisciplinary conference was held on Neonatal Intensive Care. The twenty participants approached the common topic with their various backgrounds and expertise—pediatrics, nursing, economics, social welfare, psychology, law, philosophy, and theology. Following the conference, ethicists Albert R. Jonsen and Michael J. Garland wrote an attempted synthesis of the group's ethical convergence.[53] In addition to affirming the inherent moral worth of every infant and the various stewardship responsibilities of parents, physicians, and the State for the well-being of that child, Jonsen and Garland propose the medico-moral principle, "Do no harm, without expecting compensating benefit for the patient." They conclude that life-saving or sustaining efforts should be considered harmful to the infant:

(1) "who cannot survive infancy";

(2) "who will live in intractable pain";

(3) "who cannot participate even minimally in human experience."

The authors go on to say that the first category is a synonym for infants "already in the dying state," born with irreparable lesions incompatible with life. While care remains obligatory, further prolonging efforts are counter-productive and harmful. The second category is self-explanatory. Attempts to alleviate pain, even those which may indirectly hasten death, are judged in the patient's best interest. Pain inflicted on an infant who is fundamentally incapable of fathoming a meaning for it is to be seen as unmitigated harm. Finally Jonsen and Garland define minimal participation in human experience in language akin to that used by McCormick, Johnson, Paris, et al.—"that the infant has some inherent capacity to respond affectively and cognitively to human attention and to develop toward initiation of communication with others."[54]

Caution is counseled lest "costly," "unproductive," and "unattractive" lives too facilely be equated with this category. "Protection of the most vulnerable" remains a societal keystone.

That, plus a realization of the possible fallibility of medical prognoses, calls for a conservative interpretation of this third criterion. At this point Jonsen and Garland part company with McCormick. While McCormick categorically rejects active euthanasia or direct infanticide as a viable moral option, Jonsen and Garland see it as theoretically permissible, though practically fraught with dangers and open to potential abuse.

Up to this point the quality of life proponents surveyed, in their effort to remain patient-centered, have focused primarily and/or exclusively on the patient's individualistic and physiological abilities to mentally receive or respond to sensory input. If that neurological capacity is non-existent or short-circuited by pain or burden, then treatment is non-obligatory. What factors, if any, **other than** the patient's relational capabilities and tolerance for pain, are permissible in determining a life to be inordinately burdensome to the patient?

Approximately 200,000 newborns each year pass through the Neonatal Intensive Care Units of U.S. hospitals. The estimated length of stay is from eight to eighteen days, with thirteen being the national median. One prominent neonatologist estimates that the cost per diem for treatment in a well-equipped NICU hovers near $2,000. In 1986 the national investment in neonatal intensive care ran close to $3 billion.[55] A study done a decade ago calculated the then cost of lifetime institutionalization for a single severely handicapped child to exceed $400,000.[56] John Paris cites the atypical case of a 27 year-old "decerebrate, quadriplegic" woman whose long-term (18 years) maintenance in a community hospital setting is conservatively estimated to have cost her family and/or society $6,104,590.[57] At the risk of sounding mercenary, is the financial burden placed on one's family or the society-at-large ever sufficient to warrant foregoing potentially life-saving treatment? Certainly the ordinary/extraordinary means tradition allowed cost of treatment to impact on the calculation of one's overall burden. While newborns incur no personal financial debt, the burden or cost of care **to others,** especially one's family, has traditionally been a component of burden-to-benefit balancing.

Nor is financial "cost" the sum and substance of burden that a severely handicapped child may inflict on parents, fellow siblings, and the society. In addition to depleting a family's monetary resources, a tragically deformed or diseased infant may emotionally overtax the coping resources of parents and fellow siblings. Divorces, mental breakdowns, and child behavioral problems are not uncommon in the home of a severely handicapped child. Are these potentially extraordinary psychological "costs" valid factors in the burden-to-benefit calculus?[58]

To declare treatment optional on the grounds that it represents **excessive** burden to a particular family unit is not the same as declaring it optional any time a family does not want a "defective" newborn, or wishes to avoid lifestyle infringements, or "prefers" to spend its finite resources for things other than the medical care required by a handicapped child. Rather, to regard treatment as optional for social considerations is to acknowledge "that some cases of congenital anomaly are so complicated medically and require such unusual expense and emotional involvement on the part of parents that the continued existence of the family unit is itself placed in serious jeopardy."[59] To save a child by destroying his/her social milieu is arguably not in that patient's holistic best interest.

While in theory Veatch, Arras, McCormick, Paris, et al. are willing to consider familial and social "costs" in determining the burden component related to prolonging life, ultimately their fears of potential abuse lead to non-inclusion or at least a tendency toward exclusion of such social burden factors. For example, in dealing with non-competents, Veatch rejects the general argument of "burden to others" as a legitimate reason for refusing treatment.[60] He is actually a bit ambiguous in the reasons behind this exclusion of social factors in the cases of non-competents. Clearer is John Arras who denounces as "the rankest kind of discrimination" any treatment policy that allows parental socio-economic status to determine an offspring's right and access to life-saving care.

> Even though socially induced burdens can join forces with strictly physical disabilities to make a life excessively burdensome to its bearer, we must base our treatment decisions solely on the extent of medical disabilities. To take social factors into account is to act unjustly toward the child.[61]

In "To Save or Let Die" McCormick's absolute declaration that decisions "must be made in terms of the child's good, this alone" does not in itself forestall incorporating some social factors as they relate to the infant's holistic well-being. For that matter, his advocacy of **relational potential** as the measure of an infant's minimal interest in life-saving treatment is a family-oriented, socially-conscious criterion, at least as viewed from the patient's perspective. However, in the caveats or clarifying guidelines in McCormick and Paris' more recent treatment of the topic, they shy away from allowing "institutional or managerial reasons," such as the ability of a particular family to cope, to be brought to bear. Accordingly, to make the preservation of an infant's life depend on the personalities and emotional or financial capacities of the parents alone is an unacceptable erosion of our respect for life. "No one ought to be allowed to die simply because these parents are not up to the task."[62]

As these examples illustrate, the quality of life proponents surveyed so far **tend** toward a more individualistic, physiologically-rooted (brain-related) determination of the patient's best interest, as seen from that patient's own experiential perspective. As they see it, the psychological and material burden on one's family may exempt that particular nuclear family from bearing the full burden, but it ought not prematurely diminish the infant's generally binding right to treatment or the society's **parens patriae** obligation to augment limited familial resources. Only in the rare, perhaps even hypothetical case in which the investment of resources is perceived as a **major** threat to the Common Good would a society be able to override a relationally able child's non-absolute right to life sustenance.[63]

Of those surveyed thus far, only Paul Johnson seems more willing to regularly incorporate social factors related to a family's or a society's resource limitations, provided they are weighed in as one component "affecting the actualization of the infant's life quality potential," and not as "other" claims set over against the infant's right to health care. Such a broadening of the patient's best interests to include social factors related to his/her family and society leads to a survey of those labeled "broader interpreters" of the projected quality of the patient's life standard.

2. A Broader Interpretation

Pediatric surgeon Anthony Shaw, aware that the patient's best interest and not that of the family is and ought to remain primary, states that "a true proxy of a handicapped newborn infant would . . . try to determine the capability of the infant's leading a meaningful existence."[64] However, his definition of a "meaningful existence" is far broader than that of Arras, McCormick, Paris, et al. Shaw is skeptical that barely sapient life, with the potential for minimal relationality with one's environment, is an adequate definition of a quality of life that most patients would want **or accept** as worthwhile. Despite the difficulty of evaluating the quality of another individual's life and the meaning of that life to him/her, Shaw believes there are a number of commonly accepted variables. To synthesize these factors the author devised a quasi-mathematical formula. "This formula," Shaw insists, "by no means defines the quality of life but simply suggests a dynamic relationship among three factors (two external to the patient) which affect the quality of life."[65]

To Treat or Not To Treat

$$(N.E.) \times (H. + S.) = M.L.$$

The formula reads: one's Natural Endowments multiplied by the sum of one's Home and Societal resources equals the potential for a Meaningful Life. While suggesting a 0–10 scale for natural or physiological abilities and a 1–10 scale each for familial input and social support systems, Shaw refuses to posit a total score that would arithmetically define a life as categorically not meaningful to the patient. Below the perfectly meaningful life score of 200, Shaw declines to plot a substandard line of demarcation.

In no sense is Shaw suggesting this formula be used practically to determine whether treatment should be given or withheld from handicapped infants, but he believes it clearly points out that familial and social enhancements or inhibitions do in fact improve or diminish the quality of life to be lived. A close-knit family with a strong pro-life bias would enhance a handicapped patient's potential for human development by contrast with a fractured home plagued by financial woes or even child abuse. So also, a just society which generously contributes money, time, and talent to neonatal medicine, special education, and foster care can offset some (much?) of the disability related to one's "defective" natural endowment. It is apparent to Shaw that the extent of the child's handicap is not necessarily the sole determinant of whether the child's quality of life should be judged excessively burdensome to the patient.

In tandem with the authors previously surveyed, Shaw and the other scholars gathering at this pole of the "projected quality of the patient's life" spectrum would agree that a non-sapient life, one with no (zero) natural endowment for human relationships, is not meaningful to the patient. In the best interest of this patient treatment is contra-indicated, regardless of parental devotion and societal support. So also, a natural endowment of some limited mental capacity, if offset by intractable pain, would likewise be an indication that further treatment is not warranted.

By contrast, however, Shaw, Duff, Campbell, Lorber and Weir differ from those quality of life advocates surveyed earlier in two respects. First, these scholars are unwilling to declare pain-free life with a bare minimum of relational potential to be **de facto** meaningful to the patient and worth prolonging. Second, these scholars are less skeptical of incorporating the external factors of familial and social data into the determination of an infant's qualitative best interest. According to them, the projected quality of a handicapped newborn's life is and ought to be measured on a sliding scale of interrelated factors, not so closely restricted to biological potential and individualistic burden.

Shaw illustrates the applicability of his schema and also demonstrates its variance from the more restricted approach by dealing with a case similar to the Johns Hopkins baby—a Down's Syndrome infant with duodenal atresia. Considering life with Trisomy 21 as a "moderately low" natural endowment, he posits two differing "H. + S." combinations. If the parents have rejected the infant and if society presently offers inadequate care in a largely custodial institution, this patient's potential for "meaningful life" may reasonably be judged not worth the digestive surgery. On the other hand, if there is a loving home or good foster care awaiting this Down's Syndrome sufferer, especially if special education opportunities abound, the patient's prospects for a "meaningful life" are greatly enhanced and care would generally seem advisable. Shaw reemphasizes that decisions for or against treatment "should involve consideration of the welfare of the infant alone and should be separated from consideration of the family except inasmuch as the effect on the family itself might react unfavorably on the infant."[66] Shaw entrusts these decisions to doctors and parents deciding collaboratively, in an atmosphere of full disclosure of information, support for the family, and primary concern for the newborn's welfare. Society, through its legislatures and courts, may offer guidelines and guidance.

Yale-New Haven Medical Center pediatrician Raymond S. Duff and University of Aberdeen, Scotland, Dr. A.G.M. Campbell have published together and separately no fewer than eighteen articles over the past fifteen years dealing with decisions to cease or forego treatment of handicapped newborns.[67] In their first article, which appeared in the October 1973 issue of the **New England Journal of Medicine,** Duff and Campbell stated "that the extreme excesses of Hegelian 'rational utility' under dictatorships must be avoided." However, they are equally critical of "the uncontrolled application of medical technology" prevalent in today's society, which harms by over-treatment rather than nontreatment. Striving for a middle course, Duff and Campbell adopt a quality of life standard similar to Shaw's formula—patient-centered, yet readily open to incorporating familial and social burdens as they impact on the patient's potential. "If there is little prospect of freedom from crippling disabilities that will prevent the attainment of a personal life of meaning and quality, and a measure of independence from others, then extraordinary means to sustain or prolong life are inappropriate."[68]

Notice that the definition of a "meaningful life" has been expanded from McCormick's emphasis on the "strictest possible" interpretation of **relational potential** to a life marked by "freedom from crippling disabilities" and the capacity to achieve a meaningful personal life, including some "measure of independence." They suggest that Joseph Fletcher's "indicators for humanhood" might be a useful guide for the potential functions necessary to declare the quality of an infant's life meaningful and worth prolonging. This list, to be treated more fully in the next chapter, includes not merely some minimum mental awareness, but an I.Q. of at least 40 on a standard Stanford-Binet test, a sense of time, curiosity, and relationality, all centered around neocortical function.[69]

Prior to the inclusion of social factors, Duff and Campbell believe that severe central nervous system and/or brain disorders automatically indicate a lack of even minimal potential for a meaningful quality of life. Specific examples of such problems include infants with anencephaly, hydranencephaly, extreme forms of hydrocephalus especially if complicated by other abnormalities or CNS infection, and certain chromosome disorders such as Trisomy 13. Infants with fully documented severe brain damage following asphyxia, haemorrhage or infection might also be included in this category.[70] "At the present [1977] time" they also include children with progressive degenerative diseases of the brain, such as leukodystrophies or an infant in the terminal stages of intracranial cancer. All of these cases might similarly be judged by McCormick, Paris, Johnson, et al. as further examples of the anencephalic-like infant who lacks even minimal relational potential.

But Duff and Campbell push further into controversial or borderline cases—Trisomy 18, Trisomy 21 with complications, severe cases of myelomeningocele, and severe multiple congenital abnormalities not necessarily involving the brain. In these cases "technical criteria" based on medical data alone are insufficient to project prospects for a "meaningful life" and this patient's best interest. The psychosocial factors of familial dedication, financial and personal resources, and the availability of societal assistance (Shaw's "H" and "S" factors) must be thoughtfully reviewed and incorporated by parents and the health care team. Duff and Campbell envision staff and parents functioning as a "small community," mutually informing, challenging, and refining each other's positions in search of the patient's best interest.[71] Paralleling Shaw's analysis of two socially distinct cases of Down's Syndrome, Duff and Campbell assert:

A 'good' choice for treatment might be an infant with spina bifida who is wanted, who can be cared for in a family without excessive or coerced sacrifice and for whom the family's caring is loving and voluntary. A 'bad' choice for treatment might be a similar infant but where the parents have little or no capacity to care for their child; where the family does not want to be forced to do what they believe should not be done and where resources to help the child or the family are limited or absent.[72]

While acknowledging the potential for injustice in the latter decisions, Duff and Campbell fear **more** the potential "tyranny of sometimes cruel technology" if a "disease-oriented" approach holds sway, mandating treatment irrespective of a patient's social milieu.

In defining and discerning the newborn's best interests, Duff believes "the central (often sacred) role of the family must be acknowledged and supported" even though resulting decisions at times violate a particular religious, moral, or legal doctrine. Unavoidable conflicts will arise between the rights, needs, and desires of various parties involved. "With a sense of balance, irony, and tragedy," Duff concludes that "it is understandable, right and common that the family's interests are sacrificed to benefit the child." In this he seems to be siding with the patient-centeredness principle noted in the first section of this chapter. However, he also borders on the socially-weighted approach to be surveyed in Chapter Four when he speaks of sacrificing the infant's **prima facie** right to care to the family's desire or "right to relief from pointless crushing burdens." In acknowledging that families at times are incapable of dealing with the financial and emotional strain of caring for a severely handicapped child and that State institutions are often little more than "warehouses" or "dying bins," Duff and Campbell are not necessarily negating fundamental patient-centeredness. Rather, given the circumstantial facts that the child will not be loved and cared for, lamentable as this is, they suggest that **this** patient at **this** time is best served by a decision for nontreatment.[73]

Rooted strongly in the "informed consent" principle, Duff and Campbell join Shaw in championing the patient's point of view, seeing the "capacity to live, **as he defines living**" as the ultimate determiner. If the patient is non-competent, as with all handicapped newborns and severely brain-damaged persons, one's family and physician are entrusted to discern their charge's best interests, in the light of their own values and interpretation of the patient's prognosis for a meaningful quality of life. Given this interpretive diversity, Duff and Campbell are more willing to trust parental and physician discretion, while more restrictive quality of life advocates seek to hem in guardian autonomy within certain physiological perimeters and to exclude socio-economic concerns as much as possible.

Finally, Duff and Campbell reject McCormick's categorical exclusion of active infanticide as a viable option. Dr. Duff asserts that his "patient-oriented" philosophy of deciding care logically would allow for a choice of death by passive or active means "to permit escape from excessively cruel disease or from oppressive, dehumanizing treatment."[74] It would be **nocere** or harmful to refuse treatment for a patient because of the excessive burden of continued life and yet to leave that patient existing or living in such a limbo state. Far better, if death is not imminent or if excruciating pain cannot be abated, to actively dispatch the patient as painlessly as possible.[75]

Prominent spina bifida specialist John Lorber should also be noted as a practitioner of a broader quality of life perspective, with particular reference to myelomeningocele patients. In the first day of life, newborns with myelomeningocele are judged by Lorber on the basis of six physiological criteria:

> 1) degree of hip and leg paralysis; 2) location of the spinal lesion; 3) degree of kyphosis or scoliosis (spine curvature);

4) size of the head (sign of hydrocephalus); 5) presence of intracerebral birth injury; or 6) the presence of other gross congenital defects, such as cyanotic heart disease, ectopia of bladder, or Trisomy 21.

On the basis of one or more negative indicators Lorber would recommend withholding treatment. According to Lorber, the purpose of this policy is to give every baby a chance of full treatment, provided s/he has the "potential" to live an acceptable quality of life, defined as life "with only moderate handicaps." Such a policy likewise saves other infants, who do not have such potential, from immense suffering, "interminable operations," prolonged hospitalization, and so on.[76]

Gone is McCormick's advocacy of a "strict interpretation" of the **minimal** capacity for human relationships and in its place is a standard which defines a qualitatively meaningful life as one "with only moderate handicaps" or a life free of "interminable operations" and other long-range burdens. On the basis of lack of **relational potential** alone, Johnson exempted very few spina bifida sufferers from surgical care. On the basis of a life "with only moderate handicaps," Lorber could withhold treatment from a great deal more. To be incontinent with accompanying urinary complications, paraplegic (crutches or wheelchair-bound), or to have a major spine curvature and repeated bone fractures would all indicate, for Lorber, a life severely handicapped. Behind these physical disabilities lies Lorber's own interpretation of a quality of life worth living.[77]

In an article surveying the results of 270 consecutive cases, he asserts that one's quality of life should be consistent with self-respect, happiness, and marriage. The ability to earn one's own living in the competitive employment market and "to be self-supporting with a secure, independent place in society" are also desirable.[78] It is not clear whether the projected inability to marry or to hold a job (even if one's future could be discerned at birth) would in itself constitute a life not worth prolonging. At the very least Lorber's interpretations of quality of life need clarification and further refinement. In addition to the degree of burden **for the patient,** Lorber, like Shaw, Duff, and Campbell, frequently mentions the financial and emotional "cost" to family, health care personnel, school systems, and the community of long-term care for severely handicapped children as validating reasons for nontreatment, particularly if the patient's prognosis is "poor."

Finally, it is appropriate here to note a 1984 contribution by Oklahoma State ethicist Robert F. Weir to the nontreatment debate. His volume, **Selective Nontreatment of Handicapped Newborns,** is an ambitious project, an attempted survey and critique of the medical, legal, and ethical literature on the subject, with special emphasis on the question of infanticide. What is his own ethical stance? Where does he fit on the spectrum of the four types presented in this volume? At first glance it might appear that he belongs in the next chapter with those who deny personhood to neonates and weigh their interests off against those of others in some socially-weighted calculus. After all, Weir claims affinity with H. Tristam Engelhardt and his "social person" construct. Still, Weir openly affirms that his attribution of potential personhood and its accompanying rights to all newborns is an ontological or inherent assertion. It is based on the infant's own potential "in the normal course of his or her development" to become a full person, "rather than relying on the choice of other persons . . . to ascribe a conjectural status of personhood to a neonate who does not actually possess it."[79]

This is made firmer by Weir's advocacy of "the child's best interests" as his fundamental decision-making standard. As potential persons, neonates have a **prima facie** claim to life's protection and to appropriate medical treatment. Even in those instances when one's **prima facie** claims may be overridden by "other considerations," such considerations should have only one focal point—"the best interests of the anomalous child."[80]

According to Weir, the central question in quality-of-life positions is whether a handicapped infant "has the likelihood of a meaningful life." He contrasts this, supposedly, with the central question of his own child's best interests position—"given the possibility that a handicapped infant will not have a meaningful life by normal (non-handicapped) standards, is that life likely to represent a fate worse than death or a life worth experiencing even with the handicaps?"[81] Despite Weir's protests to the contrary, it would seem that a question concerning whether one's handicapped life is "a fate worse than death" or "a life worth experiencing" is fundamentally and categorically still a **quality** of life question. He assumes that attempts to determine quality of life are necessarily comparative with other lives and therefore discriminatory against any life deemed less than ideal. However, in reality, he himself goes on to compare the state or quality of various impaired lives in terms of the patient's benefit and burden with the state of pain-free but unproductive death. Therefore, Weir fits into this author's typology with those scholars surveyed here who advocate some projected quality of the patient's life as the measure of the person's best interest. His willingness to incorporate familial and social factors, provided there is one focal point, "the best interests of the anomalous child," makes him a broader interpreter of the projected quality of the patient's life standard, not unlike Shaw, Duff, Campbell, or Lorber.[82]

In terms of case application, Weir expands the generic lists of diseases and conditions which are either untreatable (List A) or inordinately burdensome to the patient (List B). At the same time he mentions a greater number of specific cases in which one's handicapped quality of life is diminished but still worth preserving (List C).

Projected Quality of Life

"A"

Anencephaly as well as other untreatable neurological conditions (e.g., craniorachischisis totalis, myeloschisis, massive subarachnoid hemorrhage, Chiari II malformation); infantile polycystic kidney disease; untreatable types of congenital heart disease (e.g., hypoplastic left ventricle); and multiple severe anomalies requiring repetitious efforts at resuscitation.

"B"

Hydranencephaly; Trisomy 18; Trisomy 13; Lesch-Nyhan syndrome; Tay-Sachs disease; lissencephaly; cri-du-chat syndrome; and metachromatic leukodystrophy.

"C"

Hydrocephalus; most cases of prematurity; esophageal atresia with tracheo-esophageal fistula; duodenal atresia; most cases of congenital heart disease; most cases of intraventricular hemorrhage; Trisomy 21; hyaline membrane disease; most cases of spina bifida cystica; Apert's syndrome; diaphragmatic hernia; most cases of congenital kidney disease; abnormalities of the abdominal wall; exstrophy of the cloaca; neurofibromatosis; phenylketonuria; maple syrup urine disease; homocystinuria; cystic fibrosis; congenital hypothyroidism; and others too numerous to mention.[83]

Lastly, Weir advocates active infanticide in the rarest, perhaps only hypothetical cases, in which the initial decision that further therapy is not in the qualitative best interest of the infant-patient leads to a prognosis for a slow death accompanied by "prolonged suffering." Dispatching such a patient "quickly and painlessly," according to Weir, may be ethically justified, if done solely in the best interest of the neonate so plagued.

191

"Projected Quality of the Patient's Life"—A Critique

Every live-born issue from a woman's womb, however, "normal" or severely handicapped, is to be valued by the sheer fact of being human and being alive. Each newborn is inherently a person and therefore has the right to have his/her life protected and developmental potential fostered. Regardless of the infant's inability at birth to be a moral agent, s/he is to be treated as a potential subject or an end in oneself, never solely as an object or a utilitarian means to further others' ends. Whether rooted in religious convictions about creation, stewardship, and the image of God, or philosophically derived from some humanistic sense of intrinsic dignity, these fundamental presuppositions ground both the quality of life positions just presented as well as the ordinary/extraordinary means tradition surveyed earlier.

At the same time, adoption of the principle of Totality, holistically interpreted, nuances the above **prima facie** presumption toward treatment. The best interest of a living human patient is never served by an over-emphasis on vital signs in themselves. Within time and space, one's "life" in its physiological aspects is oriented toward one's more holistic best interest. The Totality principle rightly asserts that the meaning or teleological end for which life in the physical sense exists is one's fuller human flourishing in time and space and eternal life or union with God hereafter. The principle of Totality recognizes this in medical decision making by subordinating the mandate to prolong "life" to concern for one's psychological, social and eternal well-being. One's best interest is neither reduced to vitalistic life-prolongation nor expanded to subjugate the patient to social utilitarian concerns. Rather, "projected quality of the patient's life" proponents are to be commended for their balanced anthropology and patient-centered presuppositions. Burden-to-benefit determinations are holistically-viewed, with "sheer life" rightly yielding to determinations concerning "good life" and even these being subordinate to one's interest in "eternal life."

As a criterion or standard for deciding when to forego potentially life-sustaining treatment, the projected quality of patient's life approach expands and builds upon the core components of the ordinary/extraordinary tradition. It might even be asserted that the two approaches, at least as exemplified by Richard McCormick and Warren Reich respectively, differ primarily in language, but vary little in actual content. Both approaches can be said to be "means related" in that any decision for "nontreatment" by definition is focused on whether or not to inaugurate or continue the use of some proposed means, whether life-saving or merely life-prolonging. By the same token both types are in actuality "quality of the patient's life" standards in that the Totality-rooted decision for or against treatment focuses on the kind or "quality" of life that the handicapped patient will have with versus without the proposed procedure. In those cases in which the quality of the patient's life is judged already excessively burdened and the life-sustaining devices or proposed therapies serve only "to perpetuate" such a tragic quality of the patient's life, it seems to be more a debate over semantics than of content whether one labels the standard ordinary/extraordinary means with a means restriction or openly admits that it is a projected quality of the patient's life decision.

If medical means contribute to or actually cause an excessive burden to the patient, both standards exempt the patient from using these "extraordinary means." However, if the means neither enhance nor inhibit a life quality that is already deemed extraordinarily burdensome, or perhaps experientially "meaningless," from the patient's perspective, then it seems that the phrase "projected quality of the patient's life" better captures the reason for nontreatment. The concept of "means related" seems to be superfluous. If the question is treatment versus nontreatment, obviously a treatment or a proposed means is on the floor for consideration. If used or foregone the decision may or may not hinge on the benefit/burden of that drug, piece of equipment, or proposed surgery. On the other hand, it will **always** depend on the projected quality of the patient's life and the benefit/burden such a state in life is to and for the patient, holistically considered. Therefore, with all due respect for the concern contemporary ordinary/extraordinary means proponents have against the possible linkage of quality of life decisions for nontreatment with subsequent decisions for direct infanticide [see negative cautions to follow], it would seem that on the level of treatment/nontreatment decisions, THE morally determinative component is the projected quality of life for the patient, irrespective of means causation.

For that reason, McCormick, Paris, Johnson, et al. are to be commended for opening up the ordinary/extraordinary tradition with regard to nontreatment decisions and for declaring such decisions fundamentally and primarily to be quality of life determinations. The primary advantage of a "quality of life" schema is that it puts the emphasis squarely on the kind of life the patient lives or can live, rather than implying that the focus is dependent on means in any essential sense. It links together under one rationale decisions to withhold treatment in the cases of imminently dying patients **with** the cases of non-dying patients extraordinarily burdened by the means **with** those borderline cases in which the excessive burden is due to the amalgam of "diseases" or handicaps irrespective of means.

Ramsey's "curious exceptions" of permanently non-sapient and intractably pained patients as well as Reich and Weber's inordinately burdened cases perpetuated **but not caused by** means can thereby be incorporated together under this projected quality of the patient's life criterion. If imminently dying, the brevity of time left and one's desires for how to live while dying usually outweigh any minimal biological benefit derivable from interim therapies or cumbersome artificial life-support systems. It is the kind or quality of life one will live while dying that determines the course of treatment/nontreatment. If non-dying, and if the proposed physiologically beneficial means will cause a life qualitatively overburdened by pain, by financial or psychic cost, or by inconvenience, such means are optional. Why? No one is obliged to cause an excessively burdened quality of life for oneself or others just to prolong vital signs, presuming that these harsh burdens inhibit or negate one's broader best interest. Finally, if one is not dying, but lives a life already intractably pained, inordinately costly, excessively inconvenienced, or permanently "unaware" (non-sapient and non-relational), then, like the previous example, no treatment, however life-sustaining, is in this patient's **personal**, qualitative best interest.

Finally, in the area of positive aspects, "projected quality of the patient's life" proponents, compassionately aware of the Home and Society factors championed by Shaw, defend the inalienable right of those handicapped patients whose lives are saved and sustained to the necessary long-term financial, medical, emotional, and educational aid to make the most of their "defective" potential.[84] To mandate that severely handicapped infants must be treated, as Reagan's "Baby Doe" rulings have done, while simultaneously slashing budgetary funds from social program designed to meet their post-surgical "care" needs, is a species of dualism and injustice. Paul Johnson goes so far as to suggest that the converse may be true. "The less often means of increasing life quality are made available, the more choices not to maintain life may be justified." While he notes that ethical and/or medical decisions ought not simply reflect current structures of social justice, neither ought they be made without any reference to them. Recognizing that financial and personnel resources are not unlimited, allocation decisions must be made and consequences faced honestly.[85]

After that basic endorsement of the underlying principles and synthetic methodology of the projected quality of the patient's life standard it would seem that the next step would be to adopt either the more restrictive or the broader interpretation of what qualities are essential to declare a given newborn's life worth treating and below which one could forego further efforts as presumably not in his/her best interests. However, adopting a nontreatment standard based on some measurable quality of life below which "life" is not worth sustaining or prolonging is a tricky proposition, open to honest, prudential debate, as well as possible abuse. The potential in one direction for an over-protective minimalism, or in the opposite direction for a naively high expectation of near-normalcy, can hardly be denied. Sadly, both extremes are exemplified in the projected quality of the patient's life options surveyed here.

Duff, Lorber, Campbell, and Shaw, who adopt a "broader interpretation" of what qualities are essential to declare a handicapped infant's life worth living and sustaining, seem to set the minimum standard required for treatment too high. These physicians tend toward equating one's interest in life prolongation with one's functional ability to participate fully or "well" in personal goods and human experiences. While one's future capacity to be socially independent, to hold a competitive job, and to be able to marry, as Lorber suggests, are indeed kinds or qualities of life hoped for by and for all human beings, are such ideal life potentials essential for a life to have "meaning" and "worth" to a given patient? Surely handicapped rights groups would protest. Being blind, deaf, retarded, quadriplegic, paraplegic, impotent, or handicapped in some other way may inhibit one's potential for these experiential ideals. Yet, dependence on fellow human beings for one's livelihood, joblessness or sheltered workshop employment, and celibacy ought not in themselves constitute a life "worthless," "meaningless," or not worth sustaining.

I suggest that a human life with some minimal functional ability to process one's environmental input—mirrored in apparent enjoyment of food, reaction to pain, discomfort over dirty diapers, some degree of responsiveness to cuddling (cooing, rooting, smiling, muscle relaxation), and some basic "awareness" of significant others (primary care nurse, mother)—can be said to have sufficient meaning **for the patient** to presume the **prima facie** mandate to treat. Paralleling the relational potential standard of restrictive quality of the patient's life proponents, this definition of a life of minimally meaningful quality to the patient stands in sharp contrast to the fairly sophisticated functions deemed necessary by Shaw, Lorber, et al. For example, Duff and Campbell suggest that Joseph Fletcher's fifteen humanhood traits might be helpful for determining whether one's own life has enough potential for the patient to be worth saving. Accordingly, anyone with an I.Q. below 40 (a category which includes many happy, albeit handicapped Trisomy 21 citizens) or anyone lacking the mental sophistication to balance feelings with rationality or anyone unable "to communicate" in some intelligible way thereby could be categorically excluded from treatment. Presumably such patients are excessively burdened by their very mental deficiencies and would prefer non-life (or eternal life) to their present impaired existence.

The access-to-treatment of all mentally handicapped persons on the functional scale between this broader standard espoused by Duff and Campbell and the more restrictive one espoused by McCormick, Paris, et al. are threatened by this broad, near-normalcy interpretation of a quality of life worth saving. Better to err on the side of life, presuming that relatively pain-free life with mild to moderately severe retardation is a life with some potential for mental and relational participation, than to assume, based on some potentially biased middle class expectations, that such life is so devoid of experiential "good vibrations" as to be meaningless. Thus, while allowing some leeway for honest debate as to how much functional ability is essential to declare a mentally handicapped newborn relational, experientially capable of participating in embodied human life at all, it seems discriminatory and biased to set that standard so high that obviously relational retardates would be excluded from further participation, albeit limited, in life's "higher goods."

On the other hand, while espousing, with the more restrictive interpreters, that any newborn with the barest minimal potential to relate and positively experience his/her environment has an interest in life prolongation and a claim on treatment, I am reluctant to interpret the subsequent determination of potential burden in as individualistic a manner as Arras, Veatch, and, to some extent, McCormick and Paris tend to. In their admirable effort to avoid a socially-weighted bias against a patient's own experience of burden vis-á-vis benefit, I believe the more restrictive quality of life proponents have construed the determination of excessive burden too narrowly. The ultimate decision as to whether treatment is in a given patient's total best interest ought to incorporate not only medical or individualistic (i.e., experiential) burden factors, but also broader social factors, viewed from the patient's existentially-contexted vantage point. On this level, the broader interpreters of the quality of the patient's life echo the best of the ordinary/extraordinary means tradition in their insistence that the cost, psychic strain, and degree of inconvenience born by others, a non-competent's social network, ought rightly to be factored in as part of the patient's burden, holistically considered.

Arras' assertion that such inclusion of social factors is "the rankest kind of discrimination" reflects a tendency by the more restrictive quality of life proponents to isolate the neonate, detaching him/her from the realities of social context and circumstances. His conclusion that treatment decisions must be based "solely on the extent of medical disabilities" truncates the patient's interests, bordering on the medical indications policy surveyed and critiqued earlier.[86] McCormick, Paris, and Arras seem to allow the patient's social nature to impact only to the extent that s/he has physiologically-based potential to relate with others (determining one's minimal capacity to derive **benefit** from treatment), but to reject communality when it comes to the impact the patient's condition has on one's family or society (**burden** in the fullest sense). In an effort to forestall the slippery slope to a selfish social utilitarianism on the part of burdened others, the more restrictive quality of life proponents tend to exclude social burdens altogether. Rather, would it not be truer to the wisdom of the ordinary/extraordinary means tradition and fairer to the patient viewed as a social as well as a personal being to allow familial and even societal burden into the calculus concerning a handicapped patient's best interests?

In his defense of the use of non-competent subjects in non-therapeutic medical research, McCormick eloquently argues for an assumed "solidarity and Christian concern for others" on the part of the non-competent.[87] "Sharing in sociality," infants are in some sense "volunteer-able" to help the common good, provided their own individual well-being is not thereby appreciably burdened. Why, then, do he and Paris seem to exclude similar social solidarity and familial concerns from the calculus of the patient's best interest in treatment decisions related to non-competents? First, one might argue that if familial or other social factors are allowed to overrule a relationally able infant's presumed interest in therapy, the subsequent nontreatment would indeed harm the patient left untreated. Death or a more burdened quality of life seems inevitable. Therefore, contrary to the pain-free experimentation premise, incorporation of social factors in these cases cannot help but harm the patient, at least if nontreatment and foreseen death are considered not in this infant's best interest. Second, it is not clear whether McCormick and Paris absolutely exclude all social burden factors. In their joint **America** article they assert that familial factors ought not dictate an infant's access to treatment, since behind one's nuclear family there is a second line of social support or defense, the society. They decline to speculate whether the cost of handicapped care ever exceeds a society's (finite) resources or the demands in justice for its equitable distribution.

While it is questionable whether social burdens in and of themselves ought ever to so dominate a newborn's best interest as to negate a reasonably good prognosis if one is treated, it seems to be an over-reaction and a potential injustice to the patient to categorically exclude familial and/or wider social concerns altogether. It is possible that the exorbitant emotional and financial drain on a family and society, for an infant with only the barest minimal relational potential (e.g., severe brain damage due to prolonged asphyxia or Trisomy 13), is an extraordinary and optional burden given the extremely minimal benefit of such a practically non-sapient life condition **for the patient.** One might rightly project that s/he would not only not want to be sustained at such a personally futile quality of life, but would, as a "sharer in solidarity," also not want to so burden one's family and society for so little personal experience and benefit. As a corroborative, potentially scale-tipping element in a patient-centered benefit/burden calculus already heavily leaning toward nontreatment, factors related to one's inherent social nature and impact on others seem morally licit and admissible.

Like traversing a mine field one must tread lightly to avoid both extremes—the over-protective, physiologically-based, somewhat individualistic boundary of the restrictive interpreters as well as any glib incorporation of social concerns that might be deemed trivial, easily bearable, and more symptomatic of a selfish family or society than of a patient actually being over-burdened. To avoid potential bias against the patient, social burden factors ought to always be corroborative of existing patient burden or non-benefit, not set over against obvious benefit and minimal patient burden. With the exception of the means-related proviso, such decisions parallel the benefit/burden calculus of patient-centered factors adopted by the ordinary/extraordinary means standard, which traditionally included burden to one's family and community as an extension of the patient's own total best interests.

More work needs to be done by projected quality of the patient's life proponents across the spectrum to better hone, refine, and nuance both functionally and socially the generic boundaries of a life excessively burdened or without further experiential potential. Presently, D'Youville College professor Paul R. Johnson best exemplifies the middle ground between the restrictive and broader interpreters. From the former he adopts a **relational potential**, brain-related approach to the functional ability essential for embodied human flourishing and proceeds to clarify more specifically than McCormick et al. have as yet done who populates this category. However, he hovers closer to the so-called broader end of the spectrum in arguing that social or family considerations may over-ride the presumption for treatment in some few instances of relationally able infants. Lest this be seen as a socially-weighted calculus of contrary interests or rights, Johnson suggests integrating family or societal resource limitations into a broader concept of the best interest of the patient. If familial and societal limitations in fact do "affect the actualization of the infant's life quality potential," then they are rightful elements in the benefit/burden calculus concerning that unique patient's total best interests.[88]

At this point **two cautions** need to be raised concerning the adoption of any projected quality of the patient's life as the basis on which treatment or nontreatment hinges. Note first that a "caution," even if found telling, is not synonymous with an argument against the ethical validity of the quality of the patient's life approach to decision making. However, in the realm of public policy, such cautions may lend themselves to the adoption of a tighter legal boundary than ethics, other things being equal, would sanction.

1. The most practical, case-related caution with regard to

any quality of life medical ethic concerns the difficulty of translating what Andre Hellegers called religiously-rooted criterion into "biological criteria like signs, symptoms, IQs or lab results."[89] If one accepts **relational potential** as the measure of a life minimally worth prolonging from the patient's best interest perspective, as Varga, Childress, Beauchamp, Keyserlingk, McCormick, Paris, Nelson, Dedek, Zachary, E. Mahoney, Jonsen, and Garland tend to do, what anatomical standard will be used to declare a patient devoid of such potential? Surely, as Johnson and Arras define relationality in functional terms, it is intimately connected to the mental activity of one's brain, particularly of the midbrain (gray matter) and frontal lobes (neocortex). What neurological tests and devices are available to measure brain activity and, even more importantly, what level of neuronal function is essential for a child to have the minimal ability to relate with one's environment, especially with significant human others?

First of all, it must be acknowledged that medicine is a scientific **art**, not pure technology. As "applied" science, its diagnoses and prognoses are at best guesstimates, imprecise determinations of what probably is and projections of what might be in the future. To project the mental capacities essential to sustain relational potential in any patient suffering brain damage or dysfunction is extremely risky and "if" laden, particularly in early infancy. According to the President's Commission much of the difficulty in these cases arises from factual uncertainty. For many premature infants and for some of those with serious congenital defects, the only certainty is that without intensive care they are unlikely to survive. Little is known about how each individual will fare with treatment. "Neonatology is too new a field to allow accurate predictions of which babies will survive and of the complications, handicaps, and potentials that the survivors might have."[90]

In a 1979 article dealing with medical measurement of

brain functions, physician Barbara Manroe noted that presently "we cannot measure cognitive functions in the newborn period because we have no techniques for doing so." She suggested that we can only make predictions based on "the correlation of perinatal insults and functioning at later follow-up."[91] For example, a maturationally slow or premature infant may appropriately have an intermittently flat EEG or exhibit no elicitable reflexes, which in an older patient might be diagnostic indicators of cortical death. So also, cerebral "insults" prior to or shortly after birth (hemorrhages, infarctions) may preclude future, as yet inoperative cognitional abilities, rather than causing immediately discernible functional loss. If Manroe's data is still accurate in the mid-1980s this input makes physiologically-based determination of one's brain capacity and future relational potential difficult to project in the neonatal period. Newborns in general are not "very" animated, responsive, or cognitively dynamic, despite parental pride and assertions to the contrary.[92] Symptomatic determinations, at birth or shortly thereafter, of an infant's mental potential for self-awareness or relationality are tentative at best. Therefore, the possibility of predicting whether a given neonate is or will be capable of human interaction is a guesstimate at best.

Still, **relational potential,** however vague, refers to the embodied ability of a given patient to ingest sensory input. Simple behavioral observation, confirmed by neurological and behavioral testing over the first weeks **or months** of life, should be able to discern at least if "no" potential at all exists—anencephaly, exencephaly, **severe** collateral brain damage, **severe** Trisomy 13 or 18, **severe** asphyxia-related or hemorrhage-related brain insult, or a "permanent vegetative state." The cases of patients with greater possibility for brain development should, on the level of functional potential alone, be given the benefit of the doubt. Barring the presence of severe irremediable pain, the prognosis for an extraordinarily burdensome course of treatment, and inordinate social burden for their families or society, treatment should be given to these patients. In the case of premature infants even more time is required for an accurate prognosis because most neurological tests cannot be successfully administered until at least four to six weeks following a normal 38 to 40 week gestation period. Jonsen and Garland rightly suggest that the decision to terminate care for an infant requires "sufficient time for observation, mature assessment, and parental involvement in the decision."[93] They assert that it is more ethical, although perhaps more agonizing, to terminate care after a period of time than to withhold resuscitative measures at the moment of birth. Decisions for nontreatment in many cases may emerge only after a number of months, when the infant's mental prognosis becomes more calculable and increasingly more apparent.

Projected quality of the patient's life proponents, especially those labeled restrictive interpreters, are not unmindful of these cautions when they adopt certain minimal functional abilities as the earmark of an experientially meaningful life and then seek physiologically-based confirmations. Conscious both of the potential fallibility of medical diagnosis/prognosis and also of difficulties in measuring a neonate's mental (i.e., relational) capacities with much accuracy, the authors labeled restrictive interpreters of a patient's quality of life call for "prudent and discerning judgment" in the patient's behalf.[94] When in doubt, presume relational potential! Still, their willingness to forge ahead, making some decisions for nontreatment on the basis of careful, conservative, prudential estimates of mental dysfunction and correlative lack of relational potential is founded on the assumption that failure to do so will lead to greater abuse in terms of well-intentioned vitalistic mandates for over-treatment.

2. While it is beyond the stated scope of this dissertation to deal specifically with the question of active infanticide, it is interesting to note that Duff, Campbell, Shaw, Jonsen, Garland, Veatch, and Weir all allow, at least in theory, for the direct killing

of neonatal patients selected for nontreatment, particularly if the nontreatment decision consigns them to a slow, painful, "inhumane" dying process. If intractably pained or permanently unconscious or excessively burdened by one's quality of life itself, merciful infanticide is set forth as a more humane next step as opposed to continued nursing care, possibly accompanied by the licit "desire" (not necessarily a moral intention) for an earlier death. Does the adoption of a projected quality of the patient's life standard, unrestricted by means causation, necessarily lend itself to a pro-euthanasia posture? Broader interpreter John Lorber and more restrictive proponent Richard McCormick think not.

Dr. Lorber, who is accused of practicing subtle, barely veiled, "indirect infanticide" through his removal of nutritional support from those spina bifida infants selected out for nontreatment, rejects direct infanticide based on the wedge or slippery slope argument. If legalized, active euthanasia could become "a dangerous weapon in the hands of the State or ignorant or unscrupulous individuals."[95] Presumably then, if active infanticide were practiced only by wise, scrupulous caretakers, it would not be categorically immoral. Only the utilitarian potential for misuse and abuse seems to lead Lorber to exclude it from the nontreatment arsenal.

Richard McCormick likewise rejects direct infanticide, though his rationale for this "practically absolute" prohibition is not altogether clear.[96] If the obligation to sustain life rests ultimately on that life's experiential meaning and relational potential for the patient, it could be suggested to McCormick that once such meaning or potential ceases, there would be no essential reason to differentiate between nontreatment and direct dispatch. In fact, the latter might be preferable out of respect for the lingering person's eternal destiny and to save the patient's family futile expense and mental anguish.

Fellow Jesuit John Mahoney suggests that this is the potential danger inherent in a quality of life standard based so heavily on relational potential, rather than a sanctity of life standard that sees the obligation to treat grounded in essential personhood, irrespective of functional ability or potential. He asserts that regardless of one's experiential ability to relate with others, that patient remains a child of God, of one's family and society, and therefore a person with the rights to life and equitable treatment. Mahoney concludes, "Only if there is more to man than human relationship potential can one use that potential to justify letting die without also justifying killing."[97]

I suggest that both the contemporary ordinary/extraordinary means proponents surveyed earlier as well as quality of the patient's life advocates like McCormick do espouse an inherent right to life and to treatment for each and every newborn, irrespective of handicaps. However, the introduction of the principle of Totality implies that such a **prima facie** interest in treatment may be waived if the experiential, relational, and spiritual purposes for which one is alive have ceased or are irremediably short-circuited by pain or suffering. To forego treatment based on the lack of relational potential, as an expression of inordinate burden or of "the flame not being worth the candle," is not contingent upon a denial of essential personhood as Mahoney presumes.

Assuming then that a severely handicapped newborn, even one intractably pained or with no measurable relational potential, is still a rights-bearing person, one might still categorically defend his/her life right from directly intended assaults, either by acts of commission or omission, without necessarily mandating aggressive therapy to prolong life at such a burdened or minimal level. Thus, contemporary ordinary/extraordinary means supporters allow patients to die via nontreatment, while categorically condemning direct euthanasia. It would seem that McCormick is appropriating this same rationale, though his adoption of a proportionalist approach to the discussion of direct killing makes the distinction between direct and indirect "means" less airtight, in some sense less compelling.[98]

It is this researcher's belief that the tenacity with which contemporary ordinary/extraordinary means proponents like Warren Reich and Leonard Weber hold to the language of "means related," even in the cases in which the use of life-saving or life-sustaining means serve only to perpetuate an already inordinately burdened life, bespeaks their subtle, perhaps subconscious realization that with the open admission that the extraordinary burden may be one's quality of life itself, direct infanticide becomes at least arguably a humane action to relieve the nontreated non-terminal patient who lingers on. By linking the decision to the use of proposed means, even when such means neither cause nor increase one's already tragically burdened quality of life, at least one can claim to be dealing only with the nontreatment option vis-à-vis the means being contemplated.

A logical case can be made, based on acceptance of the principle of Totality, that in a few, rare cases of excessively burdened non-dying patients, direct infanticide would seem to be more humane, more patient-centered than merely ceasing treatment, allowing the patient to linger in such a hopeless or pathetic condition. Boston College ethicist Lisa Sowle Cahill develops this cautious pro-euthanasia rationale in two separate **Linacre Quarterly** articles, in which she argues that Pius XII's absolute deontological prohibition of euthanasia is inconsistent with his strong concern for the principle of Totality.[99] Short of social utilitarian or consequentialistic fears of societal abuse, Cahill suggests that one would be hard pressed to categorically reject some rare, perhaps even theoretical allowance of active infanticide, once one accepts quality of life determinations based on the principle of Totality.

A fuller discussion of the morality of active or direct euthanasia is beyond the scope of this book. However, the caution raised here concerning a quality of life approach to decisions to forego treatment is that the same projected qualities or lack thereof, which allow for withholding or withdrawing treatment, can likewise be argued as grounds to move from nontreatment to directly intended killing. The subsequent question, which would be appropriate for a related or succeeding volume, is whether such active killing is always and everywhere wrong. Granting the long-range potential for abuse, is the active taking of an inordinately pained or mentally "meaningless" life intrinsically immoral?

In summary, a projected quality of the patient's life approach to treatment/nontreatment decision making seems to best synthesize the logic underlying all patient-centered benefit/burden calculus. If the patient remains the quasi-exclusive focus of these decisions, an "if" disputed by the scholars to be surveyed in Chapter Four, what quality of the patient's life constitutes an existence so excessively burdened that the total best interests of the patient would be better served by nontreatment? Beware familial selfishness and a bourgeois bias against valid stewardship responsibilities. Beware mandating treatment on a patient solely on the basis of one's functional potential, as if s/he is not affected both by other physiological and psychological burdens as well as by the fortunes and foibles of one's family and society. Lastly, beware of premature medical prognoses. Contrary to the old cliché, time does **not** heal all wounds . . . or handicaps. But time does allow for fuller medical diagnoses and more accurate prognoses of the patient's personal potential. When in doubt as to the level of burden or of a newborn's potential, better to err on the side of continued life and time. Nontreatment decisions can be made beyond the neonatal period too. There is no need to rush to a precipitous judgment. Projecting the functional and social quality of a patient's life requires careful, self-effacing, prudential, patient-centered determinations.

NOTES

[1]Albert R. Jonsen et al., "Critical Issues in Newborn Intensive Care: A Conference Report and Policy Proposal," **Pediatrics** 53 (1975), p. 761; also in Albert R. Jonsen and Michael J. Garland, "A Moral Policy for Life/Death Decisions in the Intensive Care Nursery," in **Ethics of Newborn Intensive Care** (Berkeley: University of California Institute of Governmental Studies, 1976), p. 145.

[2]Richard A. McCormick, "To Save or Let Die," **America** 131 (1974), p. 8; also in **Journal of the American Medical Association** 229 (1974), p. 174.

[3]Richard A. McCormick, "Life-Saving and Life-Taking: A Comment," **Linacre Quarterly** 42 (May 1975), p. 110; McCormick, "To Save or Let Die," p. 8. All further citations from this article will be from the **America** printing cited in #2 above; McCormick, "The Quality of Life, the Sanctity of Life: A Theological Perspective," **Hastings Center Report** 8 (February 1978), pp. 34–35; McCormick, "Notes on Moral Theology: 1974," Theological Studies 36 (March 1975), p. 121; Richard A. McCormick, "Bioethics and Method: Where Do We Start?" **Theology Digest** 29 (Winter 1981), p. 311.

[4]Walter J. Burghardt, "Is Anyone Listening? Does Anyone Care?" **Hospital Progress** 54 (September 1973), pp. 74–79, 92.

[5]Lisa Sowle Cahill, "Within Shouting Distance: Paul Ramsey and Richard McCormick on Method," **Journal of Medicine and Philosophy** 4 (1979), p. 401.

[6]McCormick, "To Save or Let Die," p. 10; McCormick, "The Quality of Life, the Sanctity of Life," p. 396 in **How Brave a New World** reprint: "Concretely, if 'life' means only metab-

olism and vital processes, then what is meant by saying that this is a 'good in itself'? If that means a good to be preserved independently of any capacity for conscious experience, I believe it is a straightforward form of vitalism—an approach that preserves life (mere vital processes) no matter what the condition of the patient. One can and, I believe, should say that the **person** is always an incalculable value, but that at some point continuance in physical life offers the person no benefit. Indeed, to keep 'life' going can easily be an assault on the person and his or her dignity. Therefore, phrases such as 'the good of life in itself' are misleading in these discussions."

[7]Pius XII, "Cancer, A Medical and Social Problem," p. 48.

[8]Pius XII, Tranquilizers and Christian Morals," pp. 8–9; Pius XII, "Prolongation of Life," pp. 395–396.

[9]President's Commission, **Deciding to Forego.** p. 132.

[10]Ibid., pp. 134–135.

[11]John J. Paris and Richard A. McCormick, "Saving Defective Infants: Options for Life or Death," **America** 148 (April 23, 1983), p. 315; Jonsen et al., "Critical Issues in Newborn Intensive Care," p. 761; Jonsen, and Garland, "A Moral Policy for Life/Death Decisions," p. 145; John D. Arras, "Toward an Ethic of Ambiguity," **Hastings Center Report** 14 (April 1984), p. 26; Paul R. Johnson, "Selective Nontreatment and Spina Bifida," **Bioethics Quarterly** 3 (Summer 1981), pp. 91, 94, 97–98; John Lorber, "Ethical Problems in the Management of Myelomeningocele and Hydrocephalus," **Journal of the Royal College of Physicians** 10 (October 1975), p. 58.

[12]Arras, "Toward an Ethic of Ambiguity," p. 26.

[13]Heb 2:10; Col 1:24; I Pet 4:13; Congregation for the Doctrine of the Faith, "Vatican Declaration on Euthanasia," p. 156;

Anglican Working Party, *On Dying Well* (Church Information Office, Church House, Dean's Yard SW1P 3NZ, 1975), p. 21.

[14]John Donnelly, "Suffering: A Christian View," in **Infanticide and the Value of Life,** ed. Marvin Kohl, p. 166.

[15]Congregation for the Doctrine of the Faith, "Vatican Declaration on Euthanasia," p. 156; similar to: Pius XII, "Address to Physicians and Surgeons" (2/24/1957), **The Pope Speaks** 4 (1957/1958), pp. 33–49.

[16]For a fuller discussion of the problem of relieving pain consult Claudia Wallis, "Unlocking Pain's Secrets" **Time,** 11 June 1984, pp. 58–66; Vincent J. Collins, "Mananging Pain and Prolonging Life," in **New Technologies of Birth and Death: Medical, Legal, and Moral Dimensions,** pp. 144–149; President's Commission, **Deciding to Forego,** pp. 15–20, 32, 79–82, 277–286.

[17]Daniel C. Maguire, "Death and the Moral Domain," **The St. Luke's Journal of Theology** 20 (June 1977), pp. 205–206.

[18]Robert Weir, **Selective Nontreatment of Handicapped Newborns** (New York: Oxford University Press, 1984), p. 193; Richard M. Restak, "Newborn Knowledge," **Science** 82 (January/February, 1982), pp. 58–65.

[19]Gordon B. Avery, "The Morality of Drastic Intervention," in **Neonatology: Pathophysiology and Management of the Newborn,** 2d ed. (Philadelphia: J. B. Lippincott Co., 1981), pp. 11–14; Gordon B. Avery, quoted in the **Washington Post,** 11 March 1974, as noted in Jonsen, "Introduction: Ethics and Neonatal Intensive Care," p. 4; Dr. Clement Smith, "Neonatal Medicine and Quality of Life: An Historical Perspective," in **Ethics of Newborn Intensive Care,** eds. Jonsen and Garland, pp. 31–36; Judson G. Randolph in "Ethical Considerations in Surgery

of the Newborn," **Contemporary Surgery** 7 (December 1975), pp. 17–19.

[20]Norman Fost, M.D., "Putting Hospitals on Notice," **Hastings Center Report** 12 (August 1982), pp. 5–8; Dr. David Roy, "Issues in Health Care Meriting Particular Christian Concern— A Priority Issue: The Severely Defective Newborn," **Linacre Quarterly** (February 1982), pp. 60–80.

[21]Anthony Shaw, Judson G. Randolph, and Barbara Manard, "Ethical Issues in Pediatric Surgery: A National Survey of Pediatricians and Pediatric Surgeons," **Pediatrics** 60 (1977), pp. 588–599.

[22]I. David Todres et al., "Pediatricians' Attitudes Affecting Decision-making in Defective Newborns," **Pediatrics** 60 (August 1977), pp. 197–201: survey of Massachusetts pediatricians; Diana Crane, "Physicians' Attitudes Toward the Treatment of Critically Ill Patients," **Bioscience** 23 (August 1973), pp. 471–474; "Treating the Defective Newborn: A Survey of Physicians' Attitudes," **Hastings Center Report** 6 (April 1976).

[23]President's Commission, **Deciding to Forego,** p. 218; see also "Summary of Conclusions, pp. 2–9, 24–27; "Seriously Ill Newborns," pp. 197–229.

[24]Andrew C. Varga, S.J. "The Ethics of Infant Euthanasia," **Thought** 57 (December 1982), p. 446; John J. Paris and Andrew C. Varga, "Case of the Hopelessly Ill," **America** 151 (September 22, 1984), pp. 141–144.

[25]Tom L. Beauchamp and James Childress, **Principles of Biomedical Ethics** (New York: Oxford University Press, 1979 ed.), pp. 120ff. Not repeated in 1983 rev.

[26]Keyserlingk, **Sanctity of Life or Quality of Life in the**

Context of Ethics, Medicine, and Law (Ottawa: Law Reform Commission of Canada), p. 103.

[27]Richard A. McCormick, "To Save or Let Die," **America** 131 (July 13, 1974), pp. 6–10; **Journal of the American Medical Association** 229 (July 1974), pp. 172–176. This article subsequently has been reprinted in several sources, including McCormick, **How Brave a New World?** pp. 339–351; Thomas A. Shannon, ed., **Bioethics**, rev. (New York: Paulist Press, 1981), pp. 157–167; Tom L. Beauchamp and Leroy Walters, eds., **Contemporary Issues in Bioethics** (Belmont, Cal.: Wadsworth Publishing Co., 1978), pp. 331–337.

[28]Richard A. McCormick, "To Save or Let Die—A Rejoinder," **America** 131 (October 5, 1974), pp. 171–173; McCormick, "Questions in Bioethics," in "Notes on Moral Theology: 1974," **Theological Studies** 36 (March 1975), pp. 117–129; also in McCormick, **Notes On Moral Theology, 1965 Through 1980** (Washington: University Press of America, 1981), pp. 561–573; McCormick, "Life-Saving and Life-Taking: A Comment," **Linacre Quarterly** 42 (May 1975), pp. 110–115; Jim Castelli, "Life/Death Decisions—Interview with Moral Theologian Fr. Richard McCormick, S.J.," **St. Anthony Messenger** 83 (August 1975), pp. 33–35; McCormick, "A Proposal for 'Quality of Life' Criteria for Sustaining Life," **Hospital Progress** 56 (September 1975), pp. 76–79; McCormick, "The Judaeo-Christian Tradition and Bioethical Codes," in **Human Rights and Psychological Research,** ed. Eugene C. Kennedy (New York: Crowell, 1975), pp. 27–36; also reprinted in **How Brave a New World?** pp. 3–17; McCormick, "The Preservation of Life," **Linacre Quarterly** 43 (May 1976), pp. 94–100; McCormick, " 'Proxy Consent' and Experimentation in Children: Sharing in Sociality," **Hastings Center Report** 6 (December 1976), pp. 41–46; also in **How Brave a New World?** pp. 72–86; McCormick, "The Quality of Life, the

Sanctity of Life: A Theological Perspective," **Hastings Center Report** 8 (January 1978), pp. 30–36; also in **How Brave a New World?** pp. 383–401; McCormick and Robert Veatch, "The Preservation of Life and Self-Determination," **Theological Studies** 41 (June 1980): 290–296; also in **How Brave a New World?** pp. 371–382; McCormick, **How Brave a New World? Dilemmas in Bioethics** (Garden City, N.Y.: Doubleday and Company, 1981); rev. ed. (Washington: Georgetown University Press, 1981/85); McCormick, "Bioethics and Method: Where Do We Start?" **Theology Digest** 29 (Winter 1981), pp. 303–318; McCormick, "Life and Its Preservation," in "Notes on Moral Theology: 1980," **Theological Studies** 42 (March 1981), pp. 100–110; McCormick, "Guidelines for the Treatment of the Mentally Retarded," **Catholic Mind** 79 (November 1981), pp. 44–51; McCormick and Laurence H. Tribe, "Infant Doe: Where to Draw the Line," **Washington Post,** 27 July 1982; McCormick, "Les soins intensifs aux nouveau-nes handicapes," **Etudes** 357 (November 1982), pp. 493–502; McCormick, "Women, Newborns, and the Conceived," in "Notes on Moral Theology: 1982," **Theological Studies** 44 (March 1983), pp. 114–123, esp. 118–121; John J. Paris and Richard A. McCormick, "Saving Defective Infants: Options for Life or Death," **America** 148 (April 23, 1983), pp. 313–317; McCormick, "Notes on Moral Theology: 1983," **Theological Studies** 45 (March 1984), pp. 80–138, esp. 115–119; McCormick, "The Defective Infant: Practical Considerations," **Tablet** 238 (July 21, 1984), pp. 690–691; McCormick, "Caring or Starving? The Case of Claire Conroy," **America** 152 (April 6, 1985), pp. 269–273; McCormick, "The Best Interest of the Baby," **Second Opinion** 2 (July 1986), pp. 18–25.

[29]McCormick, "A Proposal for 'Quality of Life,' " p. 77.

[30]McCormick, "To Save or Let Die," p. 8.

[31] Ibid.

[32]Mk 12:28–34; Mt 22:34–40; Lk 10:25–28. The unique-ness and centrality of this passage is discussed more fully in Rudolf Schnackenburg, "Jesus' Decisive Action: The Concen-tration of All Religious Moral Precepts in the Great Command-ment of Love God and the Neighbor," in **The Moral Teaching of the New Testament** (New York: The Seabury Press, 1965), pp. 90–109.

[33]Paris, "Terminating Treatment for Newborns: A Theo-logical Perspective," **Law, Medicine, and Health Care** 10 (June 1982), p. 122; also by John Paris: Paris, "Withholding Life-Sup-porting Treatment from the Mentally Incompetent," **Linacre Quarterly** 45 (August 1978), pp. 237–248; Paris, "Death Dilem-mas (voluntary euthanasia)," **Christian Century** 98 (March 11, 1981), pp. 253–254; Paris, "Brain Death, Death, and Euthana-sia," **Thought** 57 (December 1982), pp. 476–483; Paris and McCormick [see McCormick n. 28]; Paris and Anne B. Fletcher, "Infant Doe Regulations and the Absolute Requirement to Use Nourishment and Fluids for the Dying Infant," **Law, Medicine, and Health Care** 11 (October 1983), pp. 210–213; Paris, "Letter to Editors," **Law, Medicine, and Health Care** 11 (October 1983), p. 231; Paris, "Right to Life Doesn't Demand Heroic Sac-rifice," **Wall Street Journal** (28 November 1983); Paris and Varga [see Varga n. 24].

[34]Ibid.

[35]Ibid.

[36] James B. Nelson, **Human Medicine** (Minneapolis: Augs-burg Publishing House, 1973), p. 19. Also appears in James B. Nelson and Jo Anne Smith Rohricht, **Human Medicine**, rev. ed. (1984), p. 21.

[37] Pius XII, "Cancer, A Medical and Social Problem," p. 48.

[38] Martin Nolan, "The Principle of Totality in Moral Theology," pp. 210–248.

[39] Arras, "Toward an Ethic of Ambiguity," pp. 31–33; John Arras takes great pains to distinguish his "relational potential standard" from McCormick and Paris, whom he accuses of stretching the patient's best interest standard "beyond the pale of its capabilities." According to Arras, the best interest standard has only one morally relevant consideration, the absence of pain. Since permanently non-sapient patients have no "consciousness," they feel no pain and therefore cease to have any subjective "interests" at all. It seems to me that Arras has discovered in secular or philosophical terms the meaning of the principle of Totality, on which McCormick and Paris base their decisions to forego treatment of non-relational patients. While the three might have an intramural debate as to whether bios is or is not a value in the abstract, their methods and conclusions are essentially the same, despite Arras' attempted differentiation. [McCormick and Paris, as believers, might add that the patient's interest does not stop at lack of relational potential, but shifts over (post-death) to a different "dimension."]

[40] McCormick, "A Proposal for 'Quality of Life,' " p. 78.

[41] McCormick, "The Preservation of Life," p. 100; McCormick, "To Save or Let Die," p. 10.

[42] Ibid.; similar ideas in Varga, "The Ethics of Infant Euthanasia," p. 446; Paul R. Johnson, "Selective Nontreatment of Defective Newborns," p. 46; President's Commission, **Deciding to Forego**, p. 219. The Commission also noted the case of Cephalodymus (one-headed twins), p. 220.

[43] Paris and McCormick, "Saving Defective Infants," p. 316.

[44] Paris and McCormick, "Saving Defective Infants," p. 316;

McCormick, "Les soins intensifs aux nouveau-nes handicapes," pp. 493–502; McCormick, "Notes on Moral Theology: 1982," p. 121; McCormick, "Caring or Starving?" pp. 269–273.

[45]John F. Dedek, "Two Moral Cases: Psychosurgery and Behavior Control; Grossly Malformed Infants," **Chicago Studies** 14 (Spring 1975), pp. 19–35; R. B. Zachary, "To Save or Let Die," **Tablet** 232 (February 1978), p. 175; Edward J. Mahoney, **Terminating Life Versus Allow to Die: A Study of Current Opinions in Law, Medicine, and Ethics** (Leuven: Katholieke University Te Leuven Dissertation, 1975); Edward J. Mahoney, "The Morality of Terminating Versus Allowing to Die," **Louvain Studies** 6 (Spring 1977), pp. 256–272. Mahoney developed a long-range consequentialism out of McCormick's original Proportionalism schema, **Ambiguity in Moral Choice**, which has since been nuanced and revised by McCormick in light of the pure "consequentialism" danger.

[46]Andre Hellegers, "Letting Deformed Newborns Die— McCormick's Approach," Unpublished Paper, Kennedy Institute File 20-5.2 (May 1974), p. 3. May have appeared in **Ob.-Gyn. News** 9 (1974).

[47]Paul R. Johnson, "Selective Nontreatment of Defective Newborns: An Ethical Analysis," **Linacre Quarterly** 47 (February 1980), pp. 39–53; Paul R. Johnson, "Selective Nontreatment and Spina Bifida," **Bioethics Quarterly** 3 (Summer 1981), pp. 91–111.

[48]Paul R. Johnson, "Selective Nontreatment and Spina Bifida," p. 100.

[49]Ibid., pp. 106–107.

[50]Beauchamp and Childress, **Principles of Biomedical Ethics** (1979 ed.), p. 122.

[51]Veatch, **Death, Dying, and the Biological Revolution,** p. 163.

[52]Robert M. Veatch, "Shall We Let Handicapped Children Die?" **Newsday,** 8 August 1982, pp. 1, 8–9. Quote from copy sent to me by R. Veatch, pp. 7–8.

[53]Jonsen and Garland, "A Moral Policy for Life/Death Decisions in the Intensive Care Nursery," in **Ethics of Newborn Intensive Care,** pp. 142–155. Can also be found as part of a longer article in Jonsen et al., "Critical Issues in Newborn Intensive Care," pp. 756–768, esp. pp. 760–764.

[54]Jonsen et al., "Critical Issues in Newborn Intensive Care," p. 762; Jonsen and Garland, "A Moral Policy," p. 148.

[55]Cynthia Cohen et al., "Familial and Social Obligations to Seriously Ill and Disabled Children," *Hastings Center Report* 17 (December, 1987), p. 25.

[56]Marcia J. Kramer, "Ethical Issues in Neonatal Intensive Care: An Economic Perspective," in **Ethics of Newborn Intensive Care,** eds. Jonsen and Garland, pp. 75–93.

[57]Paris, "Terminating Treatment for Newborns," p. 124: "Well, if one calculates at a very low rate of $300 a day, and builds in an inflation factor of 12 percent, 18 years of such care comes to $6,104,590."

[58]For a pathos-laden presentation of familial burden see Robert Stinson and Peggy Stinson, "On the Death of a Baby," **Atlantic Monthly** 244 (July 1979), pp. 64–66 + ; Robert Stinson and Peggy Stinson, **The Long Death of Baby Andrew** (Atlanta: Little, Brown, 1983).

[59]Weir, **Selective Nontreatment of Handicapped Newborns,** p. 215.

[60]Veatch, **Death, Dying, and the Biological Revolution,** pp. 133.

[61]Arras, "Toward an Ethic of Ambiguity," p. 28.

[62]Paris and McCormick, "Saving Defective Infants," p. 316.

[63]Not even considered is the possibility that the demands on a society's finite resources might be inordinate or excessive given the child's prognosis. Nor do these macroallocution discussions generally transcend the Western or first world to include the inequities of global health care distribution. When, if ever, does a handicapped newborn's needs yield as inordinate to other values, other equally just and humane demands for society's resources? [Stuart J. Kingma, "Mere Survival or A More Abundant Life," **Ecumenical Review** 33 (July 1981), pp. 257–271, with a helpful bibliography.]

[64]Anthony Shaw, "The Ethics of Proxy Consent," in **Decision-making and the Defective Newborn,** ed. Chester Swinyard, pp. 593.

[65]Ibid., p. 594.

[66]Ibid.

[67]Raymond S. Duff and A. G. M. Campbell, "Moral and Ethical Dilemmas in the Special Care Nursery," **New England Journal of Medicine** 289 (October 25, 1973), pp. 890–894; also in Beauchamp & Walters and Shannon anthologies; Duff, "Intentionally Killing the Innocent," **Analysis** 34 (1973), pp. 16–19; Beverly Kelsey, "Shall These Children Live? A Conversation with Dr. Raymond S. Duff," **Hastings Center Report** 5 (April 1975), pp. 5–9; Campbell, "Infants, Children, and Informed Consent," **British Medical Journal** 3 (1974), pp. 334–338; Duff, "On Deciding the Use of the Family Commons," in **Developmental Disabilities: Psychological and So-**

cial Implications, eds. Daniel Bergsma and Ann E. Pulver (New York: Alan R. Liss, 1976), pp. 73–84; Duff and Campbell, "On Deciding the Care of Severely Handicapped or Dying Persons: With Particular Reference to Infants," **Pediatrics** 57 (April 1976), pp. 487–493; Duff, "A Physician's Role in the Decision-Making Process: A Physician's Experience," in **Decision-making and the Defective Newborn,** ed. Chester A. Swinyard, pp. 194–219; Duff, "Deciding the Care of Defective Infants," in **Infanticide and the Value of Life,** ed. Marvin Kohl, pp. 96–101; Duff, "Patients, Families and Health Professionals," **Journal of the Medical Society of New Jersey** 75 (January 1978), pp. 43–47; Campbell and Duff, "Author's Response to Richard Sherlock's Commentary," **Journal of Medical Ethics** 6 (1979), pp. 141–142; Campbell and Duff, "Deciding the Care of Severely Malformed or Dying Infants," **Journal of Medical Ethics** 5 (June 1979), pp. 65–67; Duff, "Guidelines for Deciding Care of Critically Ill or Dying Patients," **Pediatrics** 64 (July 1979), pp. 17–23; Duff and Campbell, "Moral and Ethical Dilemmas: Seven Years into the Debate about Human Ambiguity," **Annals of the American Academy of Political and Social Science** 447 (January 1980), pp. 19–28; Duff, "Counseling Families and Deciding Care of Severely Defective Children: A Way of Coping With 'Medical Vietnam,'" **Pediatrics** 67 (March 1981), pp. 315–320; Campbell, "Which Infants Should Not Receive Intensive Care?" **Archives of Disease for Children** 57 (August 1982), pp. 569–671; Duff et al., "Deciding the Date of Defective Newborns—Letters," **Hastings Center Report** 12 (August 1982), pp. 43–44; Campbell, "The Right to Be Allowed to Die," **Journal of Medical Ethics** 3 (September 1983), pp. 136–140; Duff and Campbell, "Moral Commentaries and Tragic Choices," in **Euthanasia and the Newborn,** ed. R. C. McMillan and H. T. Engelhardt, Jr. (Dordrecht: D. Reidel, 1987), pp. 293–300.

[68]Campbell, "Which Infants," p. 570.

[69]Campbell and Duff, "Author's Response to Richard Sherlock's Commentary," p. 141; Duff and Campbell, "Moral and Ethical Dilemmas," p. 89; Joseph Fletcher, "Indicators of Humanhood: A Tentative Profile of Man," **Hastings Center Report** 2 (1972), pp. 1–4; Joseph Fletcher, "Humanness," in **Essays in Biomedical Ethics** (Buffalo: Prometheus Books, 1979), pp. 7–19.

[70]Campbell and Duff, "Author's Response to Richard Sherlock's Commentary," p. 141; parallel in Campbell, "Which Infants," p. 570.

[71]Duff and Campbell, "Moral and Ethical Dilemmas," p. 891.

[72]Campbell and Duff, "Author's Response to Richard Sherlock's Commentary," p. 141.

[73]Duff, "Counseling Families," p. 316; numerous case studies are cited in Duff and Campbell, "Moral and Ethical Dilemmas," p. 891; Duff, "A Physician's Role in the Decision-Making," pp. 488, 491; Duff, "Deciding the Care of Defective Infants," p. 97.

[74]Duff, "A Physician's Role in the Decision-Making," p. 215.

[75]Duff, "Patients, Families and Health Professionals," pp. 44–45; Duff and Campbell, "On Deciding the Care," pp. 487–492; Marvin Kohl, ed., **Infanticide and the Value of Life**; Marvin Kohl, ed., **Beneficent Euthanasia.**

[76]For the Lorber corpus see note 43 in Chapter One.

[77]It has been noted that a number of medical practitioners

too readily wrap their own personal values in the white physician's coat, setting forth their value determinations as "medical" prognoses. Weir (p. 229) suggests that Drs. Duff and Shaw, biased by their preference for higher, fuller "qualities of life," offer "unduly pessimistic" prognoses for handicapped patients who might be helped by therapy, while Surgeon General C. Everett Koop, a prominent right-to-lifer, is "unduly optimistic" in forecasting a patient's future.

[78]Lorber, "Spina Bifida Cystica," p. 856.

[79]Weir, **Selective Nontreatment of Handicapped Newborns,** p. 192.

[80]Ibid., pp. 194–195; parallels on pp. 183, 196: "No potential or actual person should be deprived of life without good reason, and in neonatal cases sufficiently good reasons for bringing about death are limited to detriment-benefit judgments made for the infant's sake."

[81]Ibid., p. 177.

[82]Ibid., pp. 196, 171. On these pages his blending of social and personal factors under the "child's best interests" umbrella seems clear. However, on page 215 he sounds as if he is willing to let familial stress serve as a claim over against the patient's perspective.

[83]Ibid., pp. 235–236.

[84]President's Commission, **Deciding to Forego,** pp. 7, 205, 228–229; Johnson, "Selective Nontreatment of Defective Newborns," pp. 42, 46–47; Jonsen and Garland, "A Moral Policy," p. 155; Jonsen et al., "Critical Issues in Newborn Intensive Care," pp. 756, 764; Philip R. Lee and Diane Dooley, "Social Services for the Disabled Child," in **Ethics of Newborn Intensive Care,** eds. Jonsen and Garland, pp. 64–74; Philip R. Lee, Albert R.

Jonsen, and Diane Dooley, "Social and Economic Factors Affecting Public Policy and Decision Making in the Care of the Defective Newborn," in **Decision-making and the Defective Newborn,** ed. Chester A. Swinyard, pp. 315–331; Eunice K. Shriver, "The Challenge of the Mentally Retarded," in **Medical Moral Problems,** ed. Robert Heyer (New York: Paulist Press, 1976), pp. 1–5.

[85]Johnson, "Selective Nontreatment of Defective Newborns," p. 47.

[86]Arras, "Toward an Ethic of Ambiguity," p. 28.

[87]McCormick, "Proxy Consent in the Experimentation Situation," in **How Brave a New World?** p. 63; McCormick, "Sharing in Sociality: Children and Experimentation," in **How Brave a New World?** pp. 87–98.

[88]Johnson, "Selective Nontreatment and Spina Bifida," pp. 94, 103–105.

[89]Hellegers, "Letting Deformed Newborns Die— McCormick's Approach," pp. 3–4.

[90]President's Commission, **Deciding to Forego,** p. 220.

[91]Barbara L. Manroe, "Ethical and Legal Considerations In Decision-Making For Newborns," **Perkins School of Theology Journal** 32 (Summer 1979), p. 5.

[92]Interview with Dr. Anne Fletcher, Director NICU, Children's Hospital National Medical Center, Washington, D.C., 16 January 1984.

[93]Jonsen and Garland, "A Moral Policy," p. 154; Jonsen et al., "Critical Issues in Newborn Intensive Care," p. 764.

[94]President's Commission, **Deciding to Forego,** p. 223; see also McCormick, "To Save or Let Die—A Rejoinder," p. 171.

[95]Lorber, "Early Results of Selective Treatment," p. 204; see also Lorber, "Selective Treatment of Myelomeningocele," p. 308; Lorber, "Ethical Problems in the Management," pp. 57–58.

[96]Richard A. McCormick, "Notes on Moral Theology: 1972," **Theological Studies** 34 (March 1973), pp. 70–74; appears in 1981 compilation, pp. 440–444. In 1973, McCormick rebutted Daniel Maguire's pro-euthanasia stance with a then consequentialistic form of his proportionalism methodology. He asserted that conventional wisdom defends the "convergence of probabilities" that in the practical order the basic human value of life would be threatened or compromised by allowing direct euthanasia of permanently comatose or intractably pained infants and others.

[97]John Mahoney, S.J. "McCormick on Medical Ethics," **Month** 14 (December 1981), pp. 410–411.

[98]Lisa Sowle Cahill, "Within Shouting Distance: Paul Ramsey and Richard McCormick on Method," **Journal of Medicine and Philosophy** 4 (1979), pp. 398–417, esp. 412–413: It is Cahill's conviction that McCormick's "practically absolute" prohibition of all direct euthanasia rests on shaky ground once long-term consequences (i.e., slippery slope fears) give way to proportionate validating reasons in the best interests of the suffering or mindless infant. If an infant's pain cannot be held at bay or if s/he is fundamentally incapable of relating with others, might not death, which is not an absolute evil in itself, be welcomed or even caused in the patient's total best interest? As Cahill states her challenge to McCormick, "If proportion justifies killing as a non-moral evil, then an absolute prohibition against direct euthanasia is possible only if the reason specified (relief of suffering) **never** justifies killing" (p. 413). If embodied life is a relative value, then Cahill finds it difficult to argue that an "intrinsic dis-

proportion" always exists between life and all other goods of the patient.

[99]Cahill, "A 'Natural Law' Reconsideration of Euthanasia," pp. 47–63; Lisa Sowle Cahill, "Comments on Euthanasia," **Linacre Quarterly** 44 (November 1977), pp. 299–300; Lisa Sowle Cahill, "Euthanasia: Continuing the Conversation," **Linacre Quarterly** 48 (August 1981), pp. 243–245.

Chapter Four

Socially-Weighted
Benefit/Burden Calculus

Regarding decisions to accept or forego treatment for a handicapped infant, physician-ethicist H. Tristam Engelhardt, Jr., asserts that "clinical and parental judgment may and should be guided by the expected lifestyle and the cost (in parental and societal pain and money) of its attainment."[1] This conclusion sounds strikingly similar to the position espoused by Drs. Shaw, Duff, Campbell, and Lorber in the previous chapter. Indeed, the scholars to be gathered together here to illustrate the fourth set of criteria join those labeled "broader interpreters" of the projected quality of the patient's life in advocating a primarily consequential or results-oriented approach. Likewise, both groups incorporate social as well as individual elements related to the infant patient's quality of life and future potential.

However, the distinction between the two, though subtle, is qualitatively major. Shaw, Duff, Campbell, and Lorber represent at most a **personal** benefit/burden analysis in which social concerns—financial cost, familial stress, and societal allocation of finite resources—are factored into the ethical equation **only** as they bear on the patient's own well-being and future best interests. By contrast, the moral philosophers and lone theologian to be surveyed and critiqued in this chapter forego this primary, almost exclusive emphasis on the patient. This fourth approach might be seen as the logical next step, the tilt of the seesaw from Duff's patient-centeredness with correlative social implications to an avowed **socially-weighted benefit/burden calculus**. Gone is the quasi-exclusive focus on the patient's best interest so basic to all three previous treatment/nontreatment standards. In its place is a benefit/burden calculus, a social utilitarianism of sorts, in which the individual best interests of newborn patients, especially those with debatable mental ability or potential, can be overridden by net social benefit.

These scholars believe that the socially-weighted calculus operative in triage medicine ought to be adopted more generally. The limits or at least scarcity of medical resources is a constant factor, not restricted to wartime or other extreme emergency. Parents, older siblings, the health care facility and staff, and the wider society all have material and psychic limits, coupled with rightful claims, that, at times, regrettably conflict with an individual patient's needs for attention. Some trade-off, a balancing of conflicting interests, however tragic, is unavoidable in a finite, material world. Proponents of this fourth treatment standard knowingly cross the threshold from a medical ethic so exclusively patient-centered as to impose potentially on the rights or desires of others to an ethic which attempts to more honestly accept and weigh conflicting claims. A patient has no absolute right to demand **all** the curative resources he or she requires. Accordingly, burdens to family or society may at times rightly over-ride the patient's individual needs.

This chapter will synthesize and critique nearly seventy sources, the neonatal decision-making corpus of seven ethicists, each of whom advocates a benefit/burden calculus in which the newborn patient's interests do **not** ultimately determine whether treatment is morally indicated or not. Two of the seven, Carson Strong and Bonnie Dreps Voigtlander, balance off the rightful claims of neonatal "persons" with and against the interests of family and society, yielding a moral "ought" based on net benefit for the greatest number. At the opposite end of the **socially-weighted benefit/burden calculus** spectrum are Peter Singer and Michael Tooley, who declare all neonates to be "subpersonal" beings, second class claimants in any communal benefit/burden analysis. In the middle of the spectrum are Mary Anne Warren and H. Tristam Engelhardt, Jr., who attempt to uphold a greater primacy for neonatal interests than Singer and Tooley allow, while at the same time not elevating these claims to the status of actual personal rights. Finally, the writings of theologian/situationist Joseph Fletcher will be presented somewhat as an addendum, a more and less refined representation of a socially-weighted benefit/burden calculus. A concluding section will attempt to cull together the threads of similarity and present a critique, both of the method and of a few case applications derived from a socially-weighted benefit/burden calculus with regard to handicapped newborns.

Benefit/Burden Calculus:
A Survey of Seven Approaches

1. Carson Strong/Bonnie Dreps Voigtlander

Carson Strong, of the University of Tennessee's Center for Health Sciences, asserts that a child's physician at times faces conflicting double duties, those of benevolence and non-maleficence to the interests of the infant patient as well as similar obligations to the interests of that patient's parents and kin.[2] He believes that the parents and family, who employ the physician for their child, are, in addition to the infant, that doctor's rightful clients, deserving some degree of consideration and advocacy in his/her medico-moral judgments. Strong concludes "that when a heavy burden would fall on the family with the survival of an impaired newborn, it is permissible to put the interests of the family above those of the infant."[3] Unlike Anthony Shaw's factoring in familial and societal burdens as one component of the equation to determine "Meaningful Existence" (M.E.) **for the patient,** Strong speaks of familial interests being set "above" or, in another place, "against" the infant's rightful concerns.

This is not to say that Strong espouses a flippant or selfish denigration of a non-competent patient's best interests. As a rule of thumb, largely for "utilitarian considerations," he believes neonatologists should serve as "infant-advocates." It is Strong's opinion that neonatologists should promote the best interests of the infant patient **except** when such life-saving actions would place "a large burden" on the family.[4] By challenging or actually denying that "the infant's interests should always be given priority" he opens up the ethical equation to a wider, socially-weighted cost/benefit analysis, especially in cases in which patient benefit, in quality of life terms, is minimal or burdened.

Focusing on the cases of very low birth weight infants, those born weighing 1,000 grams or less, Strong argues for a socially-weighted calculus balancing off the projected quality of the patient's life with "cost" effectiveness.[5] In terms of general patient prognoses he believes that statistical evidence does not support a general policy of withholding life-saving treatment from "premies." While brain damage due to hypoxia or oxygen deficiency is a tragic possibility, data indicates that 45% to 78.1% of low birth weight survivors have "a normal outcome."[6] Even those who survive with some manageable degree of mental retardation are, in Strong's estimation, persons with lives qualitatively worth living and worth saving. Generally the prospects for a healthy or at least manageably impaired life are sufficient to warrant treatment, if viewed solely from the patient's perspective.

However, cost analysis is no insignificant matter when it comes to the price tag of repeated surgeries and long-term care for the handicapped. A 1976–1978 study of one California Neonatal Intensive Care Unit indicated that the average cost of producing a survivor among premature, low birth weight babies was $46,340.[7] In 1982 dollars Strong estimates that to be $67,842. A prominent neonatologist interviewed suggests that the current daily cost of treatment in a sophisticated NICU may be as high as $2,000. Strong cites one study which estimated the national cost [in 1978] for neonatal intensive care alone at $1.5 billion annually.[8] Those initial neonatal care costs are multiplied many times over if one takes into account the expense of long term care—repeated surgeries, hospitalization, therapy, special education, family support services, and possible institutionalization. In addition to the potential drain on parental financial resources, society bears the brunt of these expenses in terms of medicaid and insurance payments as well as the cost of maintaining institutional facilities. While the price tag for these social programs is high, still services available are frequently considered inadequate.[9]

Nor is the "cost" or burden to others restricted to monetary concerns. For nearly all parents, the birth of a handicapped newborn precipitates an emotional crisis, which is characterized by a wide range of personal responses. Feelings of grief, failure, guilt, and humiliation frequently set in if parents feel it is somehow their fault that this child is "defective." Others are so shocked by the tragedy that denial, anger, or depression serves as their emotional reaction. Prospects for a lifetime devoted to remedial care for a handicapped child may give rise to death wishes toward the infant, which serve only to increase parental anxiety and guilt. Conflicting emotional responses between spouses and tension-laden disagreements as to what course of treatment to adopt frequently put a strain on their marital bond. Behavioral problems among fellow siblings are not uncommon. Restrictions on the family's ability to relocate or to travel often heighten tensions further.[10] A recent volume, **The Long Dying of Baby Andrew,** accurately chronicles the helplessness, hopelessness, and torturous burden encountered by one set of parents during the six month life span of their multiply-handicapped son.[11] Numerous studies have been done surveying the cost both in terms of dollars and in terms of psychological stress of caring for a severely handicapped child.

Strong's empathy for the plight of families so burdened leads him in some instances to tilt the utility scale in their favor. It is his opinion that at present, non-dying premature infants with the statistical prospect of a favorable quality of life ought generally to be treated. However, parental or familial inability to cope or to pay would absolve them of further personal obligation. Whether the decision for nontreatment and the responsibility for treatment should rest there or be shifted to society is a matter of some debate, even within Strong's own writings. He seems to conclude that current federal allocations are barely sufficient to warrant State custody and treatment of those handicapped infants with prospects for a sufficient quality of life, whose parents are incapable of bearing the burden. It is Strong's conviction that the State should interfere, mandating therapeutic treatment, **only if** the society is simultaneously willing to allocate the resources to assist parents and the child not merely to survive, but to develop and flourish. Should societal funds and commitment to this care be cut further or become grossly inadequate, then the parental right to refuse treatment would become more absolute in governing the final decision.[12]

Finally, in several articles dealing with euthanasia, Strong says that "irreversibly unconscious patients," newborn or otherwise, may cease to be "persons" in the sense that they cease to have any personal rights or actual embodied interest in life-prolongation. In the socially-weighted calculus, they are completely at the disposal of familial and societal interests. Presumably anencephalic infants as well as those suffering **severe** brain damage due to hypoxia fit this category. From an ethical perspective, Strong sees no problem with active infanticide of such neonatal interest-less patients.[13] He prefers to call such acts "corpumortasia," since, from his perspective, what is being terminated is a living human body, not a rights-bearing person. In Strong's schema, handicapped infants with less serious mental dysfunctions, comparable to the senile elderly, are still "persons" because they still have perceived interests, including desires to maintain health, to avoid pain, and to participate, however simply, in human relationships. The interests of these patients ought to weigh heavily, but not absolutely in any subsequent cost/benefit analysis.

In a somewhat similar approach, University of Tennessee alumna Bonnie Dreps Voigtlander combines a qualitative hedonistic theory of "the good" with an act utilitarian approach to "right acts," yielding what she calls a universalist consequentialism, in which minimizing suffering and maximizing happiness "for all concerned" is normative.[14] While not denying the personal benefit/burden claims of handicapped newborns, Voigtlander's ultimate emphasis on net social utility allows her to supersede an individual patient's best interests if, on balance, more people will benefit from that neglect or trade off.

To illustrate the operation and effectiveness of her proposed standard she briefly presents four case studies. Case number one involves a five and one-half month old infant who is blind and severely brain damaged, suffering chronic lung disease and heart trouble. Previous attempts to wean the infant from a ventilator have failed. This scenario is not uncommon with reference to premature infants born with Respiratory Distress Syndrome, also known as hyaline membrane disease. The medical-ethical question facing the parents and health care team is whether or not to forego further life-prolonging efforts. In practical terms, this would either involve one final attempt to wean the child from the ventilator, allowing nature to take its course thereafter, or establishing a "no code" policy forbidding resuscitative efforts during the infant's next respiratory and cardiac arrest.

Scholars representing all three previous types might well agree with Voigtlander that further curative efforts are optionally unwarranted, relatively futile, and not necessarily in this tragically handicapped patient's best interest. Ramsey might declare the patient irretrievably dying and conclude that such a patient ought to be allowed to die unencumbered, surrounded by human care. Means-related ordinary/extraordinary means proponents, like Connery and Weber, might judge the ventilator and accompanying NICU technology to be extraordinarily burdensome to the patient, given one's practically terminal prognosis. McCormick, Paris, and Shaw might see such an impaired quality of life as inordinately burdensome, lacking any meaningful future for the patient. Therefore, the best patient-centered option would be nontreatment. The crucial distinction between these three approaches and that of Voigtlander is her willingness to widen the locus of the ethical calculus: "It seems quite clear at this point that suffering will be minimized **for all concerned** if the infant is allowed to die."[15] [my emphasis]

Her second case illustration involves a multiply-handicapped infant, whose anomalies included "a large sack on the lower back, a withered and paralyzed arm and leg, a lopsided tongue, intestinal problems, no anus, no urinary outlet, and no discernible genitalia."[16] In addition, there were probable heart, lung, and brain complications, not yet fully diagnosed. From the first day of life the baby was intubated and frequently suctioned for respiratory congestion. It was recommended to the parents and family that nothing be done for the infant beyond regular nursing care and pain medication "since treatment would involve a series of assaultive surgeries with no hope for a near normal child." The child died on the fifth day in her mother's arms, comfortably sedated.

Voigtlander approves this decision as the most humane for all concerned. Viewing the spina bifida baby with multiple handicaps as "a mistake of nature," she catalogues the suffering of prolonged life both for the victim **and for the family.** The long and painful course of surgery and therapy for the infant, whom Voigtlander sees as having a "very poor prognosis" for "a happy life," leads her to conclude that nontreatment is in the patient's hedonistic best interest.

Along with this poor prognosis for the infant, Voigtlander projects a dim outlook for the family if treatment is inaugurated. She assumes that "healthy parents have a right to a normal child."[17] If their primary duty is to the preservation of personal, marital, and familial happiness, the burden of a spina bifida child with multiple anomalies impinges on all three. Specifically she mentions the financial resources that would necessarily be diverted from the care and education of the couple's other two children. She notes that the mother, who suffered through the pregnancy with agonizing intuitions that her baby was deformed, would be forced to endure even more mental anguish. The choice made for nontreatment appears to minimize suffering for all. "The infant will be spared a life of pain. The parents and family will grieve, but with the infant's death, life can begin to return to normality."[18] Voigtlander adds that active infanticide, which she notes is "not, now legal," would be the least painful alternative for all concerned in those cases in which the child is likely to linger or suffer greatly.

Voigtlander's third case parallels Ramsey's paradigm of an infant patient intractably pained—a year old child with dystropic epidermolysis bullosa. Such children rarely live past five years of age. Their brief lives are plagued by repeated episodes of blistering, loss of hair, buccal mucosal scarring, infection and scar formation often leading to severe deformities, dysphagia, fused digits, and retarded physical and sexual development. Visually the baby gave the appearance of a burn patient with open blisters over much of his body. Despite the doses of demaril administered for pain, the infant "screamed with pain and/or anticipation of pain" at the slightest touch. Mentally alert, he was seemingly distrustful of human interaction. Voigtlander suggests that fear and anticipation of pain if held may have contributed to this insecurity. The stress of home care was exhausting the mother and causing behavioral problems in siblings. Financial concerns were particularly burdensome since this "fairly afflu-ent" family was ineligible for much in the way of public financial aid.

If active infanticide were legal, Voigtlander leans toward that as arguably the most humane option to free all involved from a lengthy terminal vigil. However, given the legal prohi-bition as well as this particular set of parents' strongly held "pro-life" beliefs, Voigtlander appreciates their decision for contin-ued home care as situationally the best socially-weighted cal-culus. "(T)hey considered the financial and emotional stresses caused by their youngest child to be outweighed by the satisfac-tion they found in giving the best possible care to a child sent to them by God."[19] In another medically identical case, Voigtlan-der notes, parents may have found such burden overwhelming. "Then, active euthanasia would have been a clear ethical alter-native."[20] In either circumstantial schema, Voigtlander seems to place determinative ethical weight on the wishes and "cope-abil-ity" of the parents, not necessarily on the child's prognosis nor on the possibility of societal assistance.

Finally, Voigtlander discusses sketchily a case similar to the famous Johns Hopkins Case, that of a Down's Syndrome child with duodenal atresia. Prefacing her remarks with the declara-tion that no general rule can be made covering all cases of Down's Syndrome, she concludes that, all things considered, surgery would be in the qualitative best interests of all con-cerned. If the parents are incapable of coping with a child so manageably retarded, institutions or foster homes are readily available. However, Voigtlander notes that if Down's Syndrome is not the child's only permanent handicap or if the quality of institutional care would be poor, then the benefit/burden calculus might be weighted differently. Nontreatment might emerge as a net benefit for the multiply-handicapped child destined for substandard care and for the peace of mind of those who care about that child.[21]

Like Carson Strong, Dr. Voigtlander tends to give initial and, in some sense, primary consideration to the patient's holistic best interests. Neither of them uses the mere fact that the patient is an infant, and thereby not actually a competent moral agent, against that patient's claim for cure and care. However, in conflict cases, when the infant's interests encroach on the desires of affected others, both are willing to let those interests be balanced off in a socially-weighted benefit/burden calculus. Voigtlander presents the easier cases, in which the net best interests of all tend to coincide and coalesce. Strong is more willing to suggest the hard cases, in which the infant patient's rightful claims are over-ridden by the limits of a family's financial or psychic resources, or even, theoretically, by the limits of a society's ability to assist them.

Strong is also more willing to suggest that certain severely brain damaged patients may in actuality have no embodied interests to be weighed in a benefit/burden calculus. Such "nonpersons" are totally at the respectful disposal of affected others. This denigration of some human beings, however rare and however few, to subpersonal status represents the tip of an anthropological iceberg, which the next two authors adopt more fully, with radical implications for the interests of all neonatal patients.

2. Peter Singer/Michael Tooley

All three of the treatment standards surveyed in previous chapters remained so heavily patient-centered at least in part because each espoused a primarily inherent definition of the human person with a corresponding theory of inalienable rights. For example, in Chapter One a Church document was quoted, asserting:

... that the disabled person (whether the disability be the result of a congenital handicap, chronic illness or accident, or from mental or physical deficiency, and whatever the severity of the disability) is fully a human subject [a person] with the corresponding innate, sacred and inviolable rights.[22]

According to this view, something in the very essence of being genetically human, whether ordained by God or a fact of human nature itself, constitutes every member of the species a person, to be valued and cared for, irrespective of abilities or potential.

"Not so," say two Australian scholars, Monash University philosopher Peter Singer and American emigré Michael Tooley.[23] Citing the **Oxford English Dictionary** as a guide to accepted societal parlance, Australian Peter Singer defines "person" as "a self-conscious or rational being."[24] In his most complete work on the subject, **Practical Ethics**, Singer adds a third functional characteristic, autonomy, to the previously mentioned self-consciousness and rationality. For Singer, being genetically a member of the species **homo sapiens** is in itself irrelevant to the question of being a person. The prevalent Western and Christian bias, which draws a categorical and intrinsic moral distinction between "any human being" and all other living animals, is condemned by Singer [and also by Tooley] as discriminatory "speciesism."[25] "The mere fact that a being is a member of our own species does not in itself seem to be a relevant moral consideration, any more than membership of our own tribe, race, or nation could be, in itself, a justifiable ground for discrimination within our species."[26] To be not merely biologically **homo**, but truly **homo sapiens**, Singer believes a being must possess the actual ability to be aware, to reason, and to exercise free choice. He specifically lists human fetuses, all newborn babies, severely retarded individuals, and "brain dead" patients as examples of human beings who, in a functional sense, are less personal than well developed members of the animal kingdom.

In a similar manner University of Western Australia philosopher Michael Tooley proposed a slightly longer list of functional traits essential for a being's inclusion in the rights-bearing company of persons. One must actually possess or at least have previously possessed:

> 1) the ability to envision and desire a future; 2) the ability to conceptualize "self"; 3) the ability to be a conscious self, the subject of experiences; 4) self-consciousness; and 5) the capacity for further self-consciousness.[27]

In the decade and a half since Tooley first devised this list of neocortex-related functions, he has nuanced and refined his definition of "person" in the light of critics and neurological research. Aware that all sentient creatures have the capacity "to desire" and "to experience," at least to the extent of wishing to avoid pain or receive pleasure at any given moment, Tooley suggests that the **sine qua non** of functional personhood is the capacity to sustain desires across time, to be "a subject of non-momentary interests."[28] Memory of the past, coupled with desires or interests in the present, projected into the future by free choice—these are the indicators that a being is personal. In short, both Singer and Tooley equate personhood with the mental capacity to become a moral agent.

According to Tooley's survey of the scientific literature, the neuronal circuitry in the upper layers of the cerebral cortex, which is thought to be essential for higher mental functions, is not even present at birth.[29] Evidence indicates that it evolves during a postnatal period of tremendous neurophysiological development.[30] Therefore, from a neocortex-oriented, functionalist perspective, Tooley concludes that newborn infants up to the tenth or twelfth week of life are physiologically incapable of being persons.

Next, Tooley and Singer take up the question of healthy or only moderately retarded infants with the potential to develop into persons, functionally-speaking. Western society has traditionally accorded some actual rights or preferential status to these "potential persons." Tooley calls the rationale for this "the potentiality principle" and proceeds in great detail to refute the reasonableness of granting equality of rights to entities not yet capable of claiming those desire-based rights nor of exercising any conscious moral agency in concrete ethical situations.[31] Contrary to an intrinsic approach to human worth and rights, Tooley's functionalism makes it patently illogical to equate actual personal ability (being) with what is not now but may so become (to be). Actual persons may or even should weigh the utility or benefit of potential persons becoming fully personal in the "plus" column in decisions whether to treat or not treat, but such benefit is merely one element in a social mix.

Finally, Singer notes that even if healthy human non-persons (i.e., fetuses and infants) were to be accorded some middle-level, quasi-personal status, there are still human beings ("the hopelessly senile and the irreparably brain damaged"), whose non-personal lives lack even personhood potential and are thus identical in character to fellow non-rational animals.[32] Consequently newborns suffering **severe** mental handicaps would have two strikes against any claim to treatment. As non-personal beings their intrinsic and extrinsic value add up to only one component in the debit or credit column of a benefit/burden calculus. The fact that their mental handicap precludes any potential to become functioning actual persons necessarily weakens their case in any socially-weighted calculus, or, as Strong suggested, negates their claim altogether.

It is argued that while such human "non-persons," like their animal counterparts, have both intrinsic sentient worth and extrinsic "utility" to the moral community of persons, strictly-speaking, they have no inherent rights beyond the admonition against inhumane treatment (i.e., abuse) of sentient creatures. If newborns, as well as fetuses and the severely senile, lack the requisite neocortex structures and functional abilities for inclusion in the morally significant community of "persons," then in any benefit/burden calculus their non-absolute claims often yield to the interests and extrinsic desires of parents, older siblings, and society. Strong's preference for the newborn patient's interests **except** when in conflict with parental concerns yields to a presumption for parental benefit **except** if the infant happens to serve a utilitarian function for the family or society. S/he is not a person strictly-speaking, and arguably, in the first week(s) of life, has less functional ability than a mature dolphin, chimpanzee, ape, dog, or even a pig.[33] Declining to declare such exceptionally functioning animals to be persons in any actual sense, it only seems fair, from a functionalist perspective, to exclude newborns from that same rights-laden status.

Ultimately it comes down to a question of a benefit/burden calculus weighted on the side of parents and other moral agents affected by the infant non-person's life prolongation or death. Singer notes that one "extrinsic" reason which might generally tend to favor the treatment option is the fact that parents are usually bonded, affectionately attached to their offspring, even those seriously deformed. The severity of the handicap, particularly if it is mental or manifests itself facially, can, however, have an impact on this bond and the utilitarian value a given child has to his/her parents. If parents regret the child's birth and are truly burdened by the continued existence of a child with significant defects, Singer defends their right to kill the infant in the name of their own social welfare.[34]

Specifically he cites infants with severe cases of spina bifida, suffering paralysis from the waist down and permanent lack of bowel and bladder control. He notes that many such patients also are hydrocephalic, which can cause mental retardation. Singer concludes that if these conditions are irreparable, and if descriptions of the ensuing "miserable" quality of life for these infants are accurate, then ceasing further therapeutic efforts seems morally defensible, both for the sake of the suffering infant and that of his/her burdened caretakers. Barring extrinsic reasons for keeping the baby alive, he proposes direct infanticide as the most humane, consequentially-valid, moral choice. Paralleling Strong, Singer allows cost to enter here as a potential determinant of burden for family and society. Contrary to the cliché that "every human life is beyond price," he believes that a government's limited resources must be equitably distributed across a spectrum of valid social needs—health care, education, the arts, the environment, preventive medicine, and even more mundane public works like road maintenance.[35]

In between the extremes of trivial and tragic "defects," Singer mentions haemophilia and Down's Syndrome as debatable cases. He believes that either handicap alone could be sufficient grounds for nontreatment or even for direct infanticide, provided the parents would not grieve inordinately or be left childless by the loss.[36] Here Singer inserts a somewhat mechanistic sentiment concerning reproduction. If the parents are physiologically capable of conceiving and bearing a healthier, more "perfect" child, then the utilitarian value of sustaining a handicapped infant is substantially less. S/he is replaceable by a better model.

> When the death of a defective infant will lead to the birth of another infant with better prospects of a happy life, the total amount of happiness will be greater if the defective infant is killed. The loss of happy life for the first infant is outweighed by the gain of a happier life for the second. Therefore, if killing the haemophiliac [or Down's Syndrome child] has no adverse effect on others, it would, according to the total view, be right to kill him.[37]

Singer and Tooley each advocates active infanticide as the most humane and least costly solution to the cases of unwanted handicapped newborns. Direct, painless euthanasia frequently takes into account both the infant's subpersonal claim as a sentient being not to be pained unnecessarily as well as the "actual rights" of parents and society not to be burdened with an unwanted, unproductive human being. The poorer the prognosis for a life of "meaningful" quality for self and to others, the more reasonable the infanticide option becomes. As Singer states it, "killing a defective infant is not morally equivalent to killing a person. Very often it is not wrong at all."[38]

Tooley's advocacy of direct infanticide is even more succinctly phrased:

> Since I do not believe that human infants are persons, but only potential persons, and since I think that the destruction of potential persons is a morally neutral action, the correct conclusion seems to me to be that infanticide is in itself morally acceptable.[39]

3. Mary Anne Warren/H. Tristam Engelhardt, Jr.

In the middle of this spectrum of those advocating a "socially-weighted benefit/burden calculus" are two philosophers, who, like Strong and Voigtlander, are reluctant to deny the infant patient some claim or right to beneficial treatment. At the same time, like Singer and Tooley, each adopts a functional definition of persons, in which newborns, particularly those with severe brain deficiencies, fail to pass muster for inclusion as actual rights-bearers. Baylor School of Medicine professor H. Tristam Engelhardt, Jr., who has published at least twenty-three articles on the subject of personhood and treatment decision making, attempts to carve out a middle level, largely "utilitarian construct," called "social person."[40] Fetuses post-viability, newborns, and the severely senile or brain-damaged populate this category, thereby garnering some imputed non-absolute right to medical treatment. San Francisco State professor Mary Anne Warren parallels Engelhardt to the extent that she allows live-born humans with the capacity to become functionally personal to claim some admittedly conditional right to care under the label "potential person."[41] However, these imputed rights can be over-ridden, in conflict cases, by a benefit/burden calculus weighted on the side of net social gain.

Mary Anne Warren's almost exclusive focus in dealing with non-persons and "potential persons" is the fetus and her strong pro-abortion stand. She treats the question of handicapped new-borns only briefly in a page and a half postscript appended to later reprints of her 1973 article "On the Moral and Legal Status of Abortion." In this article, Warren joins Singer and Tooley in adopting a functional, neocortex-related definition of persons. Her list of essential traits includes consciousness, reasoning ability, self-motivated activity, self-concepts, and the capacity to communicate. She believes that it is patently obvious that a fetus fulfills none of the five prerequisites and is therefore a "non-person." She suggests that newborns also fail to pass muster for inclusion in the rights-bearing company of persons, functionally-considered.

And yet Warren has an intuitive sense that infants with the potential to become mentally functioning persons ought not as easily be made candidates for infanticide as she and the others believe fetuses are acceptable non-personal objects for abortion. "It is hard to deny that the fact that an entity is a potential person is a strong prima facie reason for not destroying it."[42] She goes on to assert that a preference for life-saving in the case of new-born "potential persons" need not be declared a right to life in the truly personal sense.[43] Rather she prefers to adopt the perspective that "potential people" are considered **by others** to be an invaluable resource, not to be squandered lightly. She sees this as analogous to the value society ascribes to natural resources and great works of art and the general prohibition against their wanton abuse or destruction. If parents do not want their newborn progeny, there are presently plenty of other people who would love to adopt that child as their own. To destroy or allow infants to die would deprive society at large and those prospective parents in particular of "a great deal of pleasure."

Secondly, even if the society were short on foster homes for unwanted babies, Warren believes that the majority ethos is presently in favor of tax-supported institutions to care for the abandoned or even handicapped infants in our midst. Unlike a fetus, whose very existence impinges on the freedom, happiness, and self determination of the mother, a newborn is a distinct commodity, whose adoption frees the parents of burden as clearly as would the child's death. "So long as there are people who want an infant preserved, and who are willing and able to provide the means of caring for it, under reasonably humane conditions, it is, **ceteris parabis** [sic], wrong to destroy it."[44] It follows, finally, that **if** an unwanted, perhaps "defective" infant were born into a society unwilling or unable to provide care, then its nontreatment or even destruction would be morally permissible. Beyond this Warren has not elaborated in print on questions concerning handicapped newborns.

At first glance H. Tristam Engelhardt's definition of personhood seems to parallel that of Warren, Tooley, and Singer, in that it is primarily neocortex-related. "(O)nly that which is rational, self-conscious and embodied in an animal organism counts as a human person."[45] If rationality, self-consciousness, and other brain-related abilities were the sum and substance of Engelhardt's functional personhood perspective, he might easily join Tooley and Singer in relegating the interests of neonatal patients to subpersonal, secondary status. However, Engelhardt posits "embodiment in a distinct animal organism" as at least a first step, a fundamental pre-condition for inclusion in the morally significant category of rights-bearing persons. This serves two ethical purposes. First, it allows Engelhardt, like Warren, to differentiate between the value and treatment of fetuses and infants. Second, it sets the stage for Engelhardt's "social person" construct, which imputes rightful status approaching that of actual functioning persons to all pre-rational and non-rational live-born members of the human species.

The fetus, at least prior to the point of viability, could be viewed as inextricably attached, dependent on the mother's circulatory and digestive systems for its very existence. This pre-viability fetus is arguably not a distinct animal organism with an embodiment unto itself and therefore is in no sense a person, whereas a newborn infant, however helpless and in need of care, is at least a distinct living being, embodied in six to ten pounds of physically independent flesh and blood. While not yet possessing the necessary rationality and self-consciousness required for "full" personhood, an infant fulfills at least one of Engelhardt's functional prerequisites. S/he could be labeled a quasi-person, developmentally one-third of the way there.

Engelhardt is concerned that Tooley's and Singer's outright rejection of the potentiality principle and their exclusive linkage of personhood to brain functions fail to do justice to the substantial continuity that does exist in the life of a human being from conception to the grave.[46] Revising the Aristotelian-Thomistic concept of progressive souls being infused along the developmental way, Engelhardt suggests that "personhood" and the functions associated with it are not instantaneously infused at "x" point in time, either prenatally or neonatally. Rather, there are qualitatively distinct plateaus achieved throughout gestation and life, in which a human being gradually assumes one or another personal ability. He contends that somewhere along the qualitative plateau from viability through birth a human being assumes one of the requisite traits for inclusion in the domain of actual persons, embodiment in a **distinct** animal organism. No longer essentially attached to the life source of the mother, the post-viability infant is a social "other," capable of fulfilling a role, of being useful to others as an object of pleasure, happiness, and affection. The mother-child or parent-child bond is a poignant social reality, a personal experience of great value to most parents. Although arational, the infant can smile, cry, coo, fuss, and in those basic responses play "a relatively independent role in a social matrix which is rational."[47]

In addition to the specific situational value that an infant may be to one's family, a "child" represents for society an illustrative paradigm for its broader commitments to foster the freedom and opportunity of fellow persons. If a community fails to nurture the intrinsic value and extrinsic worth of its "borderline" members who are not yet persons, are the rightful interests of the weak, the handicapped, and the less "useful" who are persons threatened? In other words, Engelhardt adopts by inference some form of the slippery slope argument in constructing his "social person" category. It is better to treat all live-born potential persons "as if" they are actual functioning persons, not only because they bring joy to the lives of their caretakers, but as a safeguard, a buffer zone, to prevent a crass social utilitarianism that would trample on the rights of older children or of weak and handicapped persons in the name of net communal benefit. "The social sense of person is a way of treating certain instances of human life in order to secure the life of persons strictly."[48]

For Engelhardt the decision to withhold or withdraw treatment from a particular handicapped infant, because of that child's status as a "social person," requires serious justifying reasons. He posits four possible socially-weighted factors favoring treatment over nontreatment as a general policy:

(1) the dignity of persons strictly is guarded against erosion during the various vicissitudes of health and disease,

(2) virtues of care and attention to the dependent are nurtured, and

(3) important social goals such as the successful rearing of children (and care of the aged) succeed.

In the case of infants, one can add in passing a special consideration

(4) that with luck they will become persons strictly, and that actions taken against infants could injure the persons they will eventually become.[49]

The first three, strictly-speaking, are wholly social concerns, having little or nothing to do with the patient as such. Only at the end, and added "in passing," is there mention of the newborn patient's condition and potential interests.

In other sources, Engelhardt focuses on this final, more patient-centered component. Respecting the parents as the primary locus of decision making, he concludes that the degree of possibility for this infant to become a fully realized "person" must be given significant weight in any calculus of net social welfare. Engelhardt compares and contrasts this "potential" with two other factors, the cost to parents and society of continued treatment and the amount of suffering involved for the infant.[50] Citing with approval recent court cases in behalf of handicapped individuals seeking damages on the grounds of tort for "wrongful life," he maintains that failure to adequately balance these latter two against one's handicapped potential may result in the "injury of continued existence."[51]

Tay-Sachs Disease and Lesch-Nyhan Syndrome are mentioned as examples of handicaps in which the symptomatic suffering and diminished potential of the infant, as well as the long term financial and psychic "cost" of care for the community, offset any net benefit in terms of the child's personhood potential.

Also mentioned are profoundly retarded babies with gross physical handicaps (left unnamed), whose potential for achieving either full personhood or even a "happy" sentient life are practically nil.[52] In these cases, the most humane treatment is nontreatment, allowing pneumonia or other medical complications to foreshorten a painful and expensive dying process.

Engelhardt's schema for deciding treatment cases is admittedly an expression of social utilitarianism.[53] The value for the society of preserving these "borderline" potential persons and the cost to others of care ultimately make or break any quasi-personal claim an infant "social person" has for care. Anencephalic babies, with no potential to achieve functional personhood, lay practically no claim on society and are thus presumed candidates for nontreatment. Infants suffering with severe, debilitating cases of myelomeningocele, however, may well have some rational potential. In these cases, the severity of the patient's prognosis and the social costs for others in terms of dollars and anxiety hold sway, despite a real but diminished patient potential. "(O)ne might argue that when the cost of cure would likely be very high and the probable lifestyle open to attainment very truncated, there is not a positive duty to make a large investment of money and suffering."[54] When asked how remote the prospect of a good or personal life must be in order not to be worth enduring the suffering and expense, Engelhardt said it is probably best, in the absence of a positive or actual duty to treat, to decide on the basis of "cost" to family and others. Even in the face of the prospect for a return to normalcy for the patient, Engelhardt suggests that, at least in theory, "very high costs themselves could be a sufficient criterion" to forego obviously beneficial treatment.

Engelhardt's advocacy of a certain cultural and situational flexibility and/or relativity precludes his speculating more specifically on generic neonatal cases.[55] The degree of retardation necessary to declare a tiny patient non-rational or incapable of self-consciousness is never clarified. Neither does he suggest any general guidelines as to what sort of expenses or what level of psychological strain constitutes an inordinate "cost" for a family or society. Obviously, some of those determinations require case-by-case calculations, but it would seem that some round numbers, perhaps in terms of I.Q. limits or percentages of income, budget, or GNP, might have been helpful outside parameters.

Engelhardt does allow for societal intervention on behalf of a newborn patient, if a rational consensus disagrees with parental interpretation either of the severity of the prognosis or of the amount of burden/cost involved.[56] At most, though, he believes society should intervene only in clear-cut cases of parental prejudice against a particular infant, which in turn erodes society's general commitment to children. In borderline cases, in which social as well as individual burden and benefit are genuinely debatable, Engelhardt prefers to trust parental discretion, since the infant's non-absolute claim to care is primarily in virtue of his/her social role and relation to those parents.

Finally, Engelhardt tends to be cautious about direct infanticide. Admitting that his "intuitive appreciation" of children may simply be "a cultural prejudice," he proceeds to defend **in practice** his prohibition of infanticide.[57] **In theory,** he acknowledges that, from a merciful patient's benefit perspective, active euthanasia of a terminally ill, suffering non-person, "all things being equal," would not only be permissible, but perhaps obligatory. His difficulty lies **in practice** with the "all things being equal" proviso. He is concerned that societally authorized infanticide might "erode" and "endanger" the role and care of children generally. Or as he states it, "even though one might have a duty to hasten the death of a particular child, one's duty to protect children in general could override the first duty."[58] The desire to forestall a painful, slower death for the one, a non-person strictly-speaking, is outweighed by the need to ensure the safety and environment for happiness of the many. In the end, the issue turns on whether sufficient procedural safeguards could be devised to allow limited active euthanasia of the dying or intractably pained. In his most recent book, **Euthanasia and the Newborn** (1987), Engelhardt seems somewhat more amenable to a carefully worded public policy allowing infanticide in what he calls this post-Christian secular age.

4. Joseph Fletcher

Ethical typologies are "artificial" constructs, rational attempts to systematically subdivide a continuum of moral approaches more or less neatly into distinct categories or "schools" of thought. Invariably typologies show their artificiality, or perhaps their inadequacy, when faced with a scholar whose breadth of vision, evolution across the years, or downright inconsistencies defy simple inclusion in one or another "camp." Such a scholar is retired University of Virginia Medical School ethicist Joseph Fletcher, the American patron of **Situation Ethics**.[59] With respect to the treatment of handicapped newborns, Fletcher's position is somewhat "slippery," at times seeming to align itself with the quality of life stance of Duff, Shaw, Lorber, or even McCormick, but more often hovering closer to the socially-weighted benefit/burden calculus associated with the scholars surveyed in this chapter.

Fletcher's situation ethics is best understood as a pendulum reaction to the overly legalistic, largely absolutist, religious ethics that preceded it, both in Catholic manualism and in Protestant biblicism. Though initially (1954) claiming that his "situationist" approach was "not naturalist, humanist, hedonist, utilitarian, or positivist," over the years Dr. Fletcher has more and more admitted his affinity with Bentham, Mill, and Moore, and their utilitarian approach to ethical decision making.[60] "Our situation ethics frankly joins forces with Mill; no rivalry here. We choose what is most 'useful' for the most people."[61] Regarding the treatment, nontreatment, or direct infanticide of handicapped new-borns, his position seems to have evolved in three stages over the decades, depending in part on whether he considers newborns, particularly those with mental deficiencies, to be rights-bearing persons or not.

In 1968 Fletcher commented on the actual case of a Tri-somy 21 baby, Philip Bard, in an article published in the **Atlantic Monthly**. The examining physician said that such infants are pe-culiarly susceptible to severe heart trouble, digestive ailments, and respiratory problems. Life would in all probability be "short," with mental development arresting at the age of two or three. [Given the fluidity of the data derivable during the neo-natal period such a prognosis was only a guesstimate, projecting the worst rather than the best possible prognosis.] The Bards de-cided to institutionalize Philip, partially in the interest of the in-fant's care and, admittedly, partially to save themselves and their other offspring undue long-term anguish. Mr. Bard confided that he would have preferred a miscarriage or a stillborn infant to this trauma. He prayed for the child's death and discussed with his son's pediatrician the merciful aspects of infanticide and allowing infants to die. A few hours after the baby's transfer to the sanitarium Philip died of "heart failure and jaundice." The reader is left with two conclusions: "Consider it a blessing" and "Oh, what a moral pity he was ever born." Commenting on this case Fletcher concluded:

> People in the Bards' situation have no reason to feel guilty
> about putting a Down's syndrome baby away, whether it's
> "put away" in the sense of hidden away in a sanitarium or in
> a more responsible lethal sense. It is sad, yes. Dreadful. But
> it carries no guilt. True guilt arises only from an offense
> against a person, and a Down's is not a person.[62]

To be a person, a human being in the rights-bearing sense, Fletcher posited self-awareness, conscious relationality, and rational initiative as functional prerequisites. Describing the birth of a Down's Syndrome infant as a "monstrous accident," Fletcher suggests that direct termination of this "sadly non- or un- or sub-human creature" is in the qualitiative best interest of all concerned. It would be a greater injustice, according to Fletcher, to waste resources "in keeping alive a Down's or other kind of idiot" that could better be invested in the life of a more normal child.[63] For Fletcher active infanticide may be likened to "post-natal abortion," just as he once called abortion "fetal euthanasia." If one may terminate the pregnancy of an unwanted fetus either because of a poor pre-natal diagnosis for the child-to-be or "simply because the patient [the mother] is strongly opposed to having a baby," then neonatal euthanasia is equally valid for similar reasons.[64]

Throughout the early 1970s Fletcher proposed various lists of humanhood indicators, not unlike those associated with the functional anthropologies of Tooley and Singer.[65] In 1972 and 1973 Fletcher published a short and a long form of an article in which he advocated twenty criteria, fifteen positive and five negative, for distinguishing personhood, human beingness in a functional sense, from mere biological membership in the human species. The fifteen essential traits are minimal intelligence, self-awareness, self-control, a sense of time, of futurity, of the past, capability to relate to others, concern for others, ability to communicate, control over existence, curiosity, changeability, a balance of rationality and feeling, an idiomorphous identity, and neocortical function. If a member of the human species must possess all or even a majority of the fifteen positive traits named in order to be considered a rights-bearing person, then all newborns fail the test. While all but the most severely mentally handicapped infants possess some neocortical function and thereby some degree of self-awareness and what could be called minimal intelligence in potentia, no infant can possibly be self-controlled, cognizant of time dimensions, in control of one's existence, or of one's reason/emotion balance. The ability to relate with and be concerned for others, to communicate, to be curious, to consciously change one's mind or conduct, and to view oneself as unique can be seen in the infant only with the passage of weeks or months, and then only in the most germinal sense.

As Fletcher's inquiry into "humanhood" or "personhood" criteria matured, he more and more focused on what he originally called the cardinal or "hinged" trait, neocortical function. If a member of the human species lacks all neocortical activity, Fletcher concludes that that **homo** is no longer **sapiens** and is not "truly human" in the personal sense.[66] The other fourteen positive traits, he asserts, are directly dependent on cerebral cortex activity. Therefore, the absence of such function, as in the case of all microcephalic and anencephalic newborns or those suffering massive prenatal or neonatal brain trauma, is indicative of non-personhood. He proposes that nontreatment or even active infanticide is theoretically in "their" best interest, if they can be said to have interests at all, and certainly in the financial and psychic best interest of family, medical facility, and society.

Notice that a subtle shift has taken place. If upper brain or neocortex function is the only **sine qua non** of human personhood and not necessarily the presence of the other fourteen traits, then most handicapped newborns, including Baby Philip Bard, are no longer "subpersonal." While their rights to life may still lose in a socially-weighted benefit/burden calculus against the interests of affected others, Fletcher seems to have narrowed the field of neonatal non-persons to include only those with severe permanent brain dysfunction.

In a 1978 article, "Pediatric Euthanasia: The Ethics of Selective Treatment of Spina Bifida," Fletcher's treatment of the handicapped newborn question reaches a third stage. He defines handicapped infants with spina bifida cystica as "the ones that slip through nature's merciful selection process." By this he means that, "happily," most such handicapped embryos and fetuses are spontaneously aborted. Fletcher believes we should "follow nature's example" in our ante-natal and post-natal selection process as well. He goes on in this article to declare that the debate as to the personhood of a neonate (or of a fetus) is not crucial to determining the advisability of therapeutic abortion, selective nontreatment, or direct infanticide. In an unusual, perhaps inconsistent shift from his earlier denial of "humanhood" or "personal" status to all or at least some infants, Fletcher asserts that birth is a "dialectical or nodal point" in one's development and that with live birth a qualitative leap is made, "the human organism becomes a person."[67] Subscribing to the Supreme Court's 1973 ruling, he concludes that ethical decisions to cease treatment or to end a malformed infant's life are quality of life questions concerning newborn persons, **not** contingent on debates as to that patient's personhood or social utility.

In another article published the same year, Fletcher laid the groundwork for "quality of life"-based decisions not to prolong these admittedly personal lives. He defined "so-called human rights" as "certain moral claims . . . that are ordinarily or commonly conceded," prima facie at best.[68] If life itself is not an absolute value and if "medicine's moral imperative and highest good is compassion and concern for human health and well-being," then he concludes that in some cases nontreatment or even direct infanticide may not only be an option, but a "moral **obligation**" in the patient's best interest.[69] Fletcher cites McCormick's "relational ability," Tooley's "self-consciousness," and his own "neocortical function" as viable candidates for determining the requisite minimal function for a life worth saving. In addition he notes that even where this minimal potential exists, it would still be moral to let or cause some babies to die if suffering proportionately outweighs potential happiness. Here he suggests Duff's "meaningful humanhood" as "a more adequate parameter."[70]

Nowhere in these later articles does Fletcher suggest overriding the infant patient's best interests for the social concerns of others, save in the extreme and somewhat exceptional case of a patient whose neocortex is non-functional, indicating a patient whose **personal** interests have ceased. While one might speculate, given his affinity with Mill's social utilitarianism, that net social benefit can and sometimes should over-ride a neonatal patient's personal rights and interests, such a conclusion is not evident in Fletcher's most recent (1978) treatment of pediatric euthanasia. In fact, he concludes by stating that "the only really serious ethical question" is: "What is the best thing to do in this case, for the particular patient?"[71] This is in sharp contrast to his earlier incorporation of numerous potentially conflictual social factors into the treatment decision making mix:

> first, the extent to which the parents are counseled; second, the parents' attitude toward the defects; third, the size or proportion of the risk in terms of a projected distribution of chances; fourth, the severity of the risk; fifth, the economic resources of the family; sixth, the welfare of other children involved, as well as the parents' physical and emotional capacity to cope.[72]

Will the real Joseph Fletcher please stand up? If his 1978 person-acknowledging, patient-centered articles actually reflect a fundamental change of position, then Fletcher rightly belongs with Duff, Campbell, Shaw, Lorber, and even McCormick as a "projected quality of the patient's life" proponent. However, if his seeming patient-centeredness is merely step one in a two stage benefit/burden calculus, and if the interests of affected others may outweigh the patient's interests, as his earlier corpus indicates, then Fletcher rightly belongs in this chapter as a both more and less consistent advocate of a "socially-weighted benefit/burden calculus."

A Socially-Weighted Benefit/Burden Calculus—A Critique

Of the four ethical types or treatment standards presented in this volume, this last one, now labeled "a socially-weighted benefit/burden calculus," has undergone the most scrutiny, criticism, and revision.[73] Earlier drafts placed primary emphasis on the "personhood" question, since the denial of actual personal dignity and corresponding human rights (i.e., personhood) to all newborns is certainly a linchpin for Tooley, Singer, early Fletcher, and, to some extent, Warren and Engelhardt as well. However, Voigtlander and, to a large extent, Strong accept no such open denial of the inherent worth and rights of neonatal patients. Still, they, like the others, do adopt a benefit/burden calculus in which the infant's interests—whether personal, potentially personal, or sub-personal—are, at best, only primary, never absolute. Other values, such as present or future social utility and the degree of burden one is for others can and, according to all seven scholars surveyed here, rightly should at times over-ride an infant patient's individual best interests.

By contrast each of the previous three chapters rested on the fundamental conviction that every living human being, regardless of functional ability or social utility, is a "person," inherently valuable, rights-laden, equal in some irreducible sense. Therefore, each of the three previously treated ethical types made the (newborn) patient's best interest the exclusive focus of nontreatment decisions, save in the rarest, perhaps only hypothetical cases when the very survival of the society itself depends on a reallocation of scarce resources. Such a pre-supposition of egalitarian, inherent personhood and the correlative, almost exclusive emphasis on the patient's personal best interest has been abandoned, at least in the cases of handicapped newborns, by the proponents of a socially-weighted benefit/burden calculus.

A socially-weighted benefit/burden calculus involves a two-step, sequentially ordered process. First, one must ask what value or worth is to be attributed to the patient in question, and on what basis. Does such a declaration of value involve corresponding rights? If so, how binding are those on others? This is the question of "personhood"—who counts, on what basis, and so what? Next, with the patient defined in terms of worth and degree of claim for resources available, one enters that patient's claim(s) into the benefit/burden calculus with the interests, claims, and possible rights of affected others. According to all the scholars presented in this chapter, an infant patient's claims, however personal or sub-personal, ought never be absolute, even if morally compelling in some cases.

Therefore, this critique will necessarily be two-tiered. First, the question of "person" will be discussed. Second, and more fundamentally, what are the merits and demerits of the shift from a virtually exceptionless emphasis on the patient's best interests to a socially-weighted benefit/burden calculus in which the interests of family and society are set "above" or, at least in conflict cases, over against those of the handicapped newborn patient?

1. Personhood

The concept of "personhood" is a slippery notion, more the result of philosophical pre-suppositions and an evaluative process than a self-evidently descriptive term. The point of calling someone a "person" is to declare that s/he is not to be treated as an object, a thing at our disposal. As a result of being declared personal, s/he is a subject, an end in oneself, deserving the respect and "rights" accorded all members of this morally significant category. There is no solitary sense of **person** that can be said to be its "whole sense," but rather a number of different components can be correlated to express personhood in the fullest sense.[74] Accordingly, the concept of person can refer simultaneously to at least three levels—what an entity is, what an entity can do, and how an entity is received. These can fairly neatly be labeled as inherent, functional, and social definitions or components of personhood. I believe that all the authors surveyed in this chapter give too little significance to the inherent or intrinsic value of human beingness, opting to hinge personal rights and corresponding moral responsibilities too heavily on one's functional potential or social utility.

For example, when Singer, Tooley, and early Fletcher use the term **person** they are referring solely to a functional notion, one centering around self-conscious, rational ability or at least the presence of the neocortical substratum necessary for such higher mental functions. "To be" personal is therefore synonymous with the ability "to do" sustained rational functions. Warren and Engelhardt adopt a similar functional definition when speaking of real or actual persons. So also Carson Strong adopts a similar functional definition of person with reference to "irreversibly unconscious patients." Depending on what neuronal circuitry is deemed essential to declare a given being rational enough to be a functional person, all beings, whether human or otherwise, who are sub-standard are by definition "non-persons," subpersonal entities with, at most, a secondary claim to medico-moral consideration.

To their credit Warren and Engelhardt refuse to let personhood status rest at this purely functional level. They assert that the mere potential for an infant to develop both the neuronal circuitry as well as the rational ability to function as a full moral agent ought to carry some weight in his/her behalf. Likewise, if a handicapped newborn is wanted, loved, and therefore of value to one's family or society at large, his/her claim for care, a right of sorts, is thereby enhanced. This constitutes an imputed status, a quasi-personhood, based on a patient's functional potential and social worth to and for others. Although not a person strictly (i.e., functionally) speaking, such infants are accorded human rights and treated "as if" persons for the sake of others.

However, there is a more basic definition or dimension of

what constitutes a being as a **person,** built on what an entity is as distinct from that living being's functional potential or social acceptability. Merely being a member of the human species whose healthy adult members are self-conscious, rational, and free ought to be sufficient to declare that being a person, essentially personal, regardless of functional deficiencies. Ideally all such persons would also possess the functional potential to become full participants in the community. Similarly one would hope that a responsible community of functioning personal beings would see in its immature, handicapped, or declining members an inherent value, an opportunity or a utility of sorts, which precedes and in some sense transcends their actual potential or social utility in a functional sense. Their very presence within the circle of personal beings would automatically lay obligations on the stronger, the wiser, and the more functionally fit to care for them.[75] "Stewardship for" rather than "denigration of" ought to be the moral imperative regarding the treatment of the least functional, least "useful" members of the moral community called persons. In short, it is not so much a question of denying the significance of mental functions or social value in ethical decision making as it is to acknowledge that there is another, more basic, rights-imputing reality—call it essence, nature, or inherent being—which makes each human patient, however functionally "defective" or socially unwanted, a person, a rights-bearing, interest-laden subject.

The mainstream of the Judaeo-Christian tradition champions this concept of the inherent dignity and worth of every living human being.[76] While some philosophical and biological debate flourishes around the status of pre-natal life, it is generally agreed by Christian scholars that from birth to death a member of the human species is a "being of moral worth," to be valued as an end, never solely as a functional or utilitarian means. Why? Because one's value is not wholly or even primarily ability-related. Created as images of God, redeemed by Christ Jesus, and continually sanctified by the indwelling Spirit, every living member of the human species is always already graced and worthy of respect. Natural endowments of stature, beauty, and physical or mental abilities are gifts to be used and developed well. However, one's basic significance does not depend on the amount of functional abilities one has been endowed with nor on how well one exercises those talents. Nor ought one's inherent right to care be based solely on one's social value to others. To do so would be to condone the discriminatory caste systems so prevalent in human societies. According to such tiered systems, to be rich, well-born, attractive, or academically brilliant is synonymous with being "better," morally more worthy of societal care.

To counter-balance such a functional and utilitarian bias, Jesus and, at its best, the Church champion a preferential option in the opposite direction, in behalf of the **anawim**, "the lost, the least, and the last" among us. No doubt handicapped newborns, with crippled bodies or damaged minds, are among the least "useful" in our midst. Still, their intrinsic worth, imparted by a merciful God, remains intact. Though they are not now and may never become actual moral agents, their dignity as persons, that is, as members of the morally significant human community, is no less real. Lack of the potential to become conscious, rational, free agents may and should color decisions made in their best interest, but this ought never be used to subvert these interests solely to extrinsic utility for the rest of us.

Nor is this belief in the inherent and abiding value of all human life restricted to Judaeo-Christian believers. Natural or humanistic philosophers can extrapolate such a principle from the fundamental human instincts for survival, self-protection, and parental responsibility. Actual functional ability to be a moral agent, coupled with acceptance into a social matrix, may be the fullest realization of human embodiment and personal life, but these ought not be the sole determiner for one's inclusion in that category of beings, usually called "persons," with moral rights to be protected and fostered. The "moral community" is wider than the "community of moral agents."

Closely related to the concept of inherent personhood is the correlative idea of inalienable rights. Contrary to Tooley's desire-ability prerequisite for the presence of a right, critic Philip Devine asserts that all humans, including pre-rational or non-rational newborns, have rights to things that they may not or even cannot functionally sustain interest in.[77] He speaks of the right of a child not to incur punishment for the treasonous crimes of a parent. The incarceration or even execution of the guilty traitor will necessarily impact **indirectly** on the child's life, but it is fundamentally and categorically unjust to **directly** harm the child for an offense s/he did not commit. The tender age and rational incapacity of the child to be culpable serve only to strengthen societal obligations to protect and not to abuse one's life. The child's right not to be penalized for parental crimes rests not primarily on one's functional ability to assert the claim, but more fundamentally on one's inherent dignity with its correlative justice-related rights.

Similarly, societies which respect the possession of private property recognize the right of a live-born offspring to inherit his/her parents' property, regardless of that infant's present inability to exercise the right or to defend it by writ or force. In fact, this **actual** right by birth, not by functional ability, is entrusted to the State for judgment and litigation in behalf of the as yet non-rational, semi-conscious, wholly dependent child-person. Tooley's inclination, reflecting Engelhardt's "social person" construct, is to say that this child does not now have an inheritance right, but "will come to have such a right when he is mature, and in the meantime no one else has a right to the estate."[78] If the child has no actual right, why hold the property in trusteeship? Surely other relatives, friends, or even the State could use such resources wisely. A socially-weighted benefit/burden calculus might even demand such a preference for the actual needs and claims of moral agents over the potential "as if" claim of a being devoid of rights. Also, why is it presumed that no related moral agent, a cousin or sister perhaps, has a "right" to claim the estate in the absence of any desire-based actual claim by the cooing newborn? One ought not seize an infant heir's estate because s/he has an **inherent** right to it, even if never fully conscious and despite the claims of more rational and desirous relatives.

Rights are essential and abiding claims, rooted in prior commitments (fidelity), societal co-responsibility (justice), and the very essence of being a morally significant being (integrity). As such, they do not require conscious moral agency on the part of the rights-bearer in order to lay claim to the respect of others. "To be" is the basis of rightful value, not "to do." Rights, like moral worth, precede and in some sense transcend functional abilities. The inherency component of "human beingness," while not sufficient to mandate aggressive therapy in all cases, is nonetheless not expendable in any anthropology that attempts to define person in a multi-dimensional, holistic sense. Being a live-born member of the human species is sufficient to declare a given patient a rightful person, even though functional ability and social utility would enhance and bring to fuller realization one's personal potential.

Functionalists like Singer and Tooley will denounce such nature-rooted preference for living human bodies as "species-ism." From their point of view, being genetically human is no more morally significant than being a member of a given race, ethnic group, or gender. As a critique of the pre-conceived human bias against the possibility of rational and therefore personal extra-terrestrial life or the as yet unproven thesis that higher animal species (primates, whales, and dolphins) may indeed be more rational, that is, functionally personal, than formerly imagined, Singer and Tooley have a point. However, as long as one is open, at least in theory, to the possibility that other species or even extra-terrestrial beings may also prove to be inherently valuable, functionally rational, and socially beloved, one need not be guilty of a speciesist bias in any exclusive or elitist sense.

It is my assertion that any definition of person (i.e., morally rightful beings) that fails to incorporate human beingness or essence as the foundational element is too narrow and, thus, discriminatory against the rights of the least developed members of the moral community. If this be speciesism, it is still preferable to functional elitism or pure social utilitarianism. Note once again that one's functional potential or social value may and, in some instances, should help determine whether a proposed therapy is in a given patient's personal best interest, holistically-considered. However, to incorporate such factors one need not deny nor undervalue the patient as person.

Three final comments relating to the personhood distinction are in order prior to a discussion of the merits or demerits of socially-weighting the benefit/burden calculus.

(a) In their impassioned efforts to allow both abortion and infanticide, it seems that Tooley and Singer fail to give enough importance to the developmental aspects of a human fetus/infant being and becoming structurally personal. Both authors are extremely casual about determining that point before which a human patient is sub-personal and presumably "killable" and after which s/he is a rights-bearing person. As Singer admits in his **Practical Ethics:**

> No attempt was made to determine the precise time at which humans in general become persons or quasi-persons. I did suggest that in view of a number of quite significant developments clustering together around ten to twelve weeks, it may be that humans become quasi-persons at about that time. This suggestion was, however, a highly tentative one.[79]

It would seem that if rationality or "being an enduring subject of non-momentary interests" is so essential to one's personal dignity and rightful status, Tooley and Singer owe it to infant patients to more carefully define when in fact they become functionally personal. It is not evident that the development of neuronal circuitry in the upper brain post-partum is necessarily a more compelling point for declaring a patient structurally rational than any of a number of brain-related developments from the early weeks post-conception onward. Nor is the presence of such neocortical circuitry synonymous with the reality of such equipment functioning rationally, actually sustaining non-momentary interests. One might as easily argue that many months pass before human children link moments into rational thought patterns. Or what about the significance of birth or viability? For Tooley and Singer those major events in one's becoming an independent bodily being seem to have no bearing at all on one's personal status. It is not my intention here to argue for another structural/functional nodal point, but merely to challenge that any lone biological conception is adequate as the hinge for determining personal worth and rights.

Likewise, though infanticide is beyond the scope of this study, Tooley and Singer leave themselves open to widespread neonatal euthanasia for any manner of reason if personhood is categorically put off until after certain post-natal brain development occurs. At the very least it would seem that Tooley and Singer ought to make some distinction between healthy, mentally normal infants enroute to "functional personhood" and those whose handicaps preclude such potential altogether. Surely the former lay at least some claim to a greater measure of care, akin to Warren's "potential persons," even if only in view of their being-on-the-way status.

Singer seems open to a hierarchy of worths with reference to the animal kingdom in that higher primates, dolphins, and some other mammals are judged to be more personal, in a functional sense, than lower species or even than some tragically deformed humans. If he can see the animal species as hierarchically spread out along the evolutionary chain, it seems a bit abrupt and somewhat prejudicial not to allow some fluidity along the human chain from conception forward. In short, even if a functional definition of person were to hold sway, one might question Tooley and Singer either for not plotting more responsibly the threshold between all animals, which have at least some "quasi-right" not to be hurt unnecessarily, and personal beings, or else for not admitting that no such hard and fast line can be determined within the developmental process of a human being and becoming more so.

(b) One might be tempted to conclude that of the seven scholars surveyed in this chapter, only five (Singer, Tooley, early Fletcher, Engelhardt, and Warren) deny or undervalue the sufficiency of ontic humanness as grounds for personal dignity and rights. Since Carson Strong and Bonnie Dreps Voigtlander seem to give primacy to the infant's best interests in their admittedly consequential calculations one might conclude that they accept membership in the human species as sufficient warrant for personal status and correlative rights. Though neither blatantly denies the **prima facie** right of newborns to claim treatment, two areas in Strong's corpus and at least one of Voigtlander's case applications give one pause.

As noted earlier, Strong declares "irreversibly unconscious patients," newborn or otherwise, to be non-persons.[80] If he honestly believes in the inherent rather than a purely functional basis for personal status, how can this be? Scholars across the spectrum admit that a permanently non-rational patient may have no further functional or personal interest in remaining alive. In that sense, nontreatment may indeed be said to be in his/her best interest. However, in order to declare such a human life personally deficient and to judge life-sustaining therapy futile in an experiential sense, one need not deny the patient's abiding worth as a person, albeit minimally equipped. Strong's denial of this abiding dignity in the case of the "irreversibly unconscious" leads me to question if his definition of who counts is not more functionally-grounded than he generally admits. At least this implies some anthropological ambiguity requiring further clarification.

In a related vein, Strong's doctoral dissertation on the relationship of informed consent and proxy consent contains a section in which he examines whether so-called "future persons" actually possess the rights to life, self-determination, and informed consent via proxy.[81] Although he clearly includes fetuses in this "future person" category, he ambiguously treats the merits/demerits of experimentation on infant subjects in the same section, implying that they as yet may only be "future persons," not rights-bearing persons in any actual sense. If this is an accurate gleaning of the texts, Strong here adopts a social construct similar to Warren's or Engelhardt's, which may impart a person-like status on potential rational beings, but which reserves real or actual personhood only for functionally self-conscious, free "subjects of non-momentary interests." Strong's use of these two subpersonal human categories leads me to believe that, at best, his affirmation of the inherent personal worth of newborn patients rests on shaky ground, perhaps more functionally-rooted and socially-motivated than it initially seemed.

Likewise, while Voigtlander never actually denies the personhood of human infants, she does tend to undervalue or at times ignore their rightful claims in her case applications. For example, in her third paradigmatic case, that of an infant suffering the blistering pain of dystropic epidermolysis bullosa, she condones nontreatment or even active infanticide as arguably in the patient's best interest. Yet, in deciding the moral course to be followed, this extraordinarily burdened state of the infant person seemingly becomes a non-factor. Parental "satisfaction" and sense of responsibility or, in the opposite scenario, parental anguish and financial burden are Voigtlander's ultimate (sole?) moral determinants. The child's right to accept or refuse treatment is subordinated **completely** to familial cares. Is this the same respect that she would accord the wishes or best interest of a functionally competent patient? Or is Voigtlander subtly allowing the supposedly personal interests of the infant patient to be denigrated and with them that patient's personhood status as well?

Voigtlander's assertion that "healthy parents have a right to a normal child" also potentially assaults the counter-vailing personhood and rights of a handicapped child born into such a hostile environment.[82] If the understandable parental desire to have a normal, healthy child becomes an actual right, as Voigtlander implies, then all unhealthy and abnormal newborns have room to fear for their continued existence. I not only challenge Voigtlander's "right to a normal child" premise, but I suggest that such an assertion and her ready advocacy of direct infanticide may bespeak a weaker sense of neonatal personhood than one might assume at first glance.

(c) Notwithstanding all these reservations about the undervaluing or denial of personal status for newborns, especially those with serious mental handicaps, the scholars surveyed here do rightly raise a counter-vailing point to the "inherency" bias of those who might be called rigorous "pro-lifers" of the vitalistic variety. To be a person, a rights-bearing being with a claim to life and equitable health care, it is enough to be a living member of the species whose competent adults are self-conscious, rational, and free-willed. However, sufficiency is not the measure of one's well-being or best interest. To be fully personal one hopefully can do those things which functionally differentiate realized persons from persons in potentia. So also, to be fully personal is to be interrelational, loving and beloved in a social network of rightful others.

Thus, Singer, Tooley, Warren, Engelhardt, Strong, Voigtlander, and early Fletcher are correct in bringing functional ability and social utility to bear on treatment questions. Vitalistic or rigorous right-to-lifers have an unfortunate tendency to canonize the biological component human life, mandating life-saving therapy irrespective of the presence or absence of these higher, fuller personal dimensions. On the other hand, the seven scholars surveyed here regrettably swing the pendulum too far in the functionalist/utilitarian direction, in an attempt to offset this vitalism or human speciesist bias. Neither extreme serves the best interest of the human patient, who is essentially to be valued, functionally to be enhanced, and always socially contexted. It seems that, in terms of case applications, contemporary proponents of the ordinary/extraordinary means tradition as well as some advocates of the projected quality of the patient's life approach do a better job of upholding the inherent dignity and rights of all patients, while at the same time remaining open to the impact that functional disabilities and heavy social burden may have on the advisability of future therapeutic efforts.

2. "Socially-Weighted" Calculus

While the espousal of a functionally-biased anthropology is the preliminary element in the treatment standard proposed here, THE universally professed component common to all seven is their willingness to over-ride a given newborn patient's individual interests in the name of a socially-weighted benefit/burden calculus. The qualitative benefit and burden of treatment for a given patient is placed on the ethical scale **over against** the benefit (utility) and burden of said treatment and patient for the community of affected persons. If the latter social concerns coalesce with the former patient-centered claims, then the patient wins, either receiving the beneficial treatment or else being spared the agony of excessively burdensome, even futile efforts. However, if life-prolonging, even qualitatively beneficial therapy, will inordinately tax that patient's family or society, it is then in **their** best interests, and thus morally justified, to withhold or withdraw treatment. For some, active infanticide would be the most humane, efficient, and least costly next step. Even in the face of the prospect for a return to normalcy for the patient, Engelhardt suggests that, at least in theory, "very high costs themselves could be a sufficient criterion" to cease obviously beneficial treatment.[83]

In this section and the critique sections of previous chapters I have advocated a holistic concept of the infant patient and of his/her best interests. Given that, the major criticism made of Ramsey's medical indications policy was precisely that it tends to reduce the scope of the (non-dying) handicapped newborn's best interest too narrowly to the physical reality of a pumping, living human organism. To their credit, both the contemporary proponents of ordinary/extraordinary means and the "broader interpreters" of the projected quality of the patient's life widen the scope of the patient's best interest to include psychological and spiritual as well as social factors, all under the principle of Totality.

In that light, the scholars gathered here under the rubric of a socially-weighted benefit/burden calculus are similarly to be commended for incorporating social factors into any ethical equation concerning individual patients. To isolate a newborn patient as if s/he is a monad wholly unrelated to family, society, and their incarnate limitations is to create an ahistorical, unreal setting for decision making. Macro-allocation questions concerning budgetary priorities in light of the limits of global resources lead to valid ethical questions concerning whether any patient, generically-speaking, has a right to soak up an inordinate and unjust share of health care dollars, talent, and energy. If the potential benefit for the patient or a category of patients is significantly diminished by the severity of the handicap, the question of relatively futile use of resources becomes even more poignant.

One need only look briefly and somewhat sketchily at some of the financial statistics to realize that the Northern/Western World absorbs an incredible proportion of the planet's resources in its quest for therapeutic medical cures. In the quarter century since 1960, health care expenditures in the United States alone have risen 1250%, reaching $356 billion for the single year 1983.[84] The percentage of that annual total which goes for care of the chronically ill and handicapped is always disproportionate to their percentage in the general patient population. For example, in 1981 the 2.2 million Americans with chronic disorders (3.8% of all patients treated that year) accounted for 20% or one-fifth of all hospitalizations and nearly 10% of all clinical visits, percentages far beyond their statistical numbers.[85] As Carson Strong noted, the initial NICU costs for handicapped newborn survivors, which he averaged at $67,842 per patient for 1982, are merely the tip of an expensive iceberg that extends beyond the neonatal period, perhaps for a lifetime. It includes not only repeated medical treatments (surgeries, hospitalizations, diagnostic testing, and physical therapy), but a battery of costly social services as well (counseling for patient and parents, special education, support services, and, for some, institutional living facilities).

The very fact that one can even talk about expenditures up to hundreds of thousands of dollars for one newborn patient is contingent on a Western or Northern, first world environment, complete with health insurance, medicaid, and/or socialized medicine. On a global scale this prompts largely unexplored macro-allocation and distributive justice questions concerning the vast amounts of money and medical resources invested in extraordinary and frequently experimental therapies for the severely afflicted few in the industrialized hemispheres, while literally millions of Africans may starve to death for want of ordinary bread and simple medical care.[86] Viewed from a global distributive justice standpoint or situationally from a hut in some third world village, the options and obligations to treat become far more complicated and/or limited.

If money and resources were limitless, it would seem ghoulish to even suggest setting price restrictions on the amount of treatment to be offered. As it is, however, the scholars surveyed in this chapter join those surveyed in Chapters Two and Three in rightly raising the specter of how much expenditure is too much. When, in the name of the equitable distribution of limited resources, do we say that what can be done need not or perhaps ought not be done?

There is a subtle but important distinction between socially-weighting macro-allocation questions on a societal, public policy level and suggesting that same method for bedside/cribside decision making. In the former, a socially-weighted calculus may of necessity be operative to determine societal priorities, the most equitable approach to distributing limited resources among a plurality of rightful claims and categories of recipients. In a sense, deciding macro-allocation questions with reference to scarce medical resources prescinds from and prefaces actual medical practice. Society, through its legislatures and philosophical systems, sets parameters on what resources are actually available for patients, physicians, and families about which to make treatment decisions.

One cannot flippantly presume that society at large can or ought to pick up the health care slack in every case of an overly taxed patient or family. The macro-allocation questions cited above indicate that the national "family" and the global "community" disperse **limited** resources as well. Given the finitude of societal funds and the necessity of prioritizing needs for those resources, it may become necessary to categorically exclude some dollar amounts or certain inevitably expensive species of cases. No individual patient, however personal and in need, has an absolute right to all resources. Therefore, in theory, a socially-weighted benefit/burden calculus, in those extreme "beyond the limits" cases, is understandable and ethically defensible. Even the scholars surveyed in Chapters One through Three at times seem to allow for a socially-weighted calculus, though only in the rarest, somewhat hypothetical cases, in which the very survival of one's society or of the moral community is at stake (war, plague, or enduring famine).

On this public policy plane, **prior to** the decision making dilemma regarding a particular physician, a circumstantially-contexted set of parents, and a unique neonatal patient, a socially-weighted benefit/burden calculus may well be the best moral course for settling macro-allocation disputes. For example, the wartime triage practice of depriving more severely wounded soldiers of their "fair share" of a scarce drug in order to give massive, healing doses to troops less severely hurt and more likely to rejoin their regiments is deemed "just" in the name of the larger war effort, even if inequitable to a given category of rightful patient-persons. Similarly, one might advocate a massive shift of health care talent and dollars to the starving peoples of Ethiopia or the Sudan at the risk of understaffing or underequipping a "state of the art" N.I.C.U. or oncology unit in an American health care facility. Unfortunately, some few grossly premature infants or massively-tumored cancer victims might die for lack of that shifted funding, expertise, and energy.

No easy resolutions of such priority debates exist. The prudential nature of such judgments calls for a careful system of checks and balances, perhaps through advocacy groups, to ward off potential bias. In the end, a socially-weighted macro-allocation calculus, while not ideal, is perhaps a necessary method for determining the Common Good, the most equitable public distribution of regrettably limited resouces among the mix of needs and classes of rightful persons.

However, once one enters the arena of actual medical practice, "intra-system" as it were, advocacy of a socially-weighted benefit/burden calculus becomes a dangerous threat to the integrity, personhood, and rightful place that has always been reserved for the individual sick or handicapped patient in need. Carson Strong's assertion that a handicapped infant patient's family is also and perhaps equally the physician's client is categorically false, at least according to the Hippocratic medical tradition. The **Hippocratic Oath** appears to be wholly patient-centered, asking physicians to vow: "Whatever houses I may visit, I will come for the benefit of the sick, remaining free of all intentional injustice. . . . "[87] No mention is made of the conflicting interests of the patient's family and no license is given to over-ride "the benefit of the sick" in the name of benefit or burden to others **considered precisely as "other."** The ordinary/extraordinary means tradition ushered in the possibility of expanding the notion of the patient-person and of his/her best interest to include such social components as cost and burden to affected others, but always as subsidiary elements of the patient's interests, holistically-considered, never as distinct counter-claims.

Thus, the EXCLUSIVE focus in actual medical practice and related decision making has heretofore always been on the best interest(s) of the patient, however broadly defined. To shift that focus toward a socially-weighted calculus in which the patient's rightful interests are merely one component among a series of presumably equal counter-claims is to undervalue the primacy of the patient and to potentially discriminate against his/her rights and best interests.

Few parents would say, all things being equal, that they "want" a physically or mentally impaired offspring. For that matter, few handicapped persons would say that, given a choice, they would still "want" to be blind, deaf, retarded, paraplegic, etc. However, with birth there is no guarantee of bodily wholeness. Contrary to Voigtlander's assertion, healthy parents do **not** have a "right" to a "normal" or "perfect" child. Parents do, nonetheless, have a responsibility, in stewardship, to protect, foster, and safeguard the inherent rights of the fruit of their womb. In most cases parents and physicians do tend to put the best interest of the newborn patient first and foremost. Parental love and the Hippocratic tradition generally combine to highlight and foster this focus on the patient's well-being. However, the birth of a severely handicapped infant, or of one not so severely damaged but whose disfigurement is particularly grotesque, often wreaks havoc on this benevolent instinct. Revulsion, guilt, shock—all those understandable emotional responses outlined by Strong—may take over, clouding one's judgment and sense of parental responsibility. It is at those junctures that potential discrimination looms largest and the rights of the handicapped newborn person are most in need of structural safeguards.

It is in these tragic cases that a holistic, patient-centered ethic, one which attempts to incorporate valid social factors of familial stress and financial limits **from the patient's perspective,** serves as a buffer zone against selfish, perhaps transitory, and unjust bias. On the other hand, it is in these same tragic instances that a socially-weighted calculus may act as a wedge, which lends itself to the further denigration of neonatal patients in the name of functional anthropologies or pure social utility. A socially-weighted calculus, however reasonable and well-intentioned, tends to undervalue the patient, particularly if that patient is mentally "substandard" and not competent to defend his/her own interests. Add to this the fact that all seven scholars surveyed here by definition denigrate the inherent worth and rightful status of newborns and other non-competent patients and the case is made stronger that a socially-weighted calculus applied within medical practice greases the slippery slope toward bias against and abuse of those patients least able to assert their rights and needs in the decision making debate.

In order to safeguard the abiding personhood and correlative "access to treatment" right of the less functional and least useful among us, a patient-centered medical ethic gives exclusive primacy to the patient's best interests. Except for the generic boundaries placed on available health care resources by society on the macro-allocation level, all specific case applications ought to incorporate social factors from the patient's perspective, as valid elements in a broader concept of the patient's personal (i.e., holistic) best interests.[88]

In this light, Strong's admirable concern for a particular family, whose financial and psychic capacities have been stretched by the demands of a severely handicapped newborn beyond its ability to cope, is not overlooked. If the society can absorb the infant's costs and medical demands within its admittedly finite health care parameters, then the infant's rightful needs oblige the community to act as extended family, provided further care offers the handicapped patient reasonable benefit without inordinate burden. However, if neither the society nor the family has the psychic or financial wherewithal to continue the infant's care, then it might be preferable to expand our concept of the infant's total best interest to include the burden of his/her care on significant others as an element in determining that patient's net burden/benefit, rather than setting those social factors or resource limits over against our primary locus, the patient-person. This is obviously more a prudential judgment call, a question of how best to prioritize and interrelate "social" vis-à-vis "individual" factors, than a question of dichotomizing the two.

It should be noted that the seven scholars surveyed here tend to shun socially-weighting the calculus when dealing with competent patients making treatment/nontreatment decisions. If the patient is functionally rational, his/her interpretation of personal best interest is given controlling weight, under the principles of self-determination and informed consent. While Singer argues that such an absolutizing of the autonomy principle may serve as a safeguard for the rights of persons in general, thus a socially-weighted value, it is usually defended in the name of functional personhood and correlative rights attached irrevocably to that privileged status.[89] A double standard seems to be operative, in which the personhood proviso treated earlier is inextricably linked with the subsequent willingness or unwillingness of these authors to socially-weight the decision making calculus. Given this potential of a socially-weighted calculus to denigrate the inherent personhood and inalienable rights of disabled and non-competent patients, changing the centuries-old focus of medicine from patient cure and care to a social utilitarianism of sorts, one should reject such a medical ethics model on the treatment/nontreatment decision-making level.

Finally, some brief mention should be made of the specific case applications proposed in this chapter. In several instances, such as Voigtlander's cases in which excessive burden for the individual patient tends to coalesce with related burdens to one's family, I would concur with the option for nontreatment, with the proviso that the latter social concerns be viewed as a corroborative element of the patient's own burden. Accordingly, the severely brain-damaged R.D.S. baby (Case #1) and the infant with severe untreatable spina bifida (Case #2) both may be judged excessively burdened and further treatment optionally contra-indicated. This, however, is not intended to condone Voigtlander's easy advocacy of direct infanticide as the most efficient and humane next step. Her presentation of the infant with epidermolysis bullosa, as noted earlier, is less clear because she tends to discount her initial assertion that the patient is in a state of irremediable pain and proceeds to acquiesce solely to the feelings of obligation or rejection on the part of the parents. On the contrary, it would seem that parental dedication or revulsion ought to be a secondary, subsidiary element in determining this tragically afflicted patient's best interests. The child-patient's pain and mental anguish ought to remain the primary factor in determining whether further life-prolonging effort is a net benefit to him/her. Patient-centered factors of physiological and psychological burden ought never be "ignored," even in those instances when a reasonable judgment about social burden may impact on the determination of the patient's holistic well-being.

Engelhardt mentions infants with Tay Sachs disease and Lesch-Nyhan syndrome as potential candidates for nontreatment, given the terminal nature of these anomalies, their gross symptoms in later stages, and the inevitable burden such children are for their families. In my judgment somewhere along the course of treatment from relatively normal birth through death at the age of four or five one ought to call a halt to further, increasingly futile therapies, if possible to forestall the child's having to cope with the worst of the disease-related symptoms. However, as with the Voigtlander examples, it would be preferable to concentrate exclusively on the infant's benefit and burden, allowing familial stress to impact as one component among many involved in determining at what point, from the patient's perspective, further efforts tilt the scale from beneficial to burdensome, from presumably desired to understandably optional.

What I reject is any denigration of the patient's worth or personhood based on his/her failure to meet some functional, brain-related standard. Tooley, Singer, and early Fletcher openly espouse such functional concepts of person, which by definition subjugate any interest "non-personal" neonates may have to the concerns of affected "persons." Paradigmatic is early Fletcher's comment concerning Baby Philip Bard: "that in dealing with Down's cases it is obvious that the end everybody wants is death."[90] Fletcher's categorical exclusion (in this source) of Down's Syndrome infants from the company of "persons" and his consequential defense of direct infanticide of such unwanted newborns as the best means to put them away **for all concerned** illustrates clearly the threat to all handicapped persons of a functional definition of person, especially when combined with a socially-weighted calculus. Aside from the fact that all Trisomy 21 children are rightful persons, most even from a neocortex-related functionalist perspective, one must disagree with Fletcher's presumption that life with or for most Down's children is undesirable. Many children with Trisomy 21 are famously mild mannered, extremely trusting, and, despite some manageable burdens, often a joy for their family and loved ones. Down's Syndrome children obviously place some burden on others not necessarily experienced in rearing a more "normal" child, but that is not and ought not be grounds to presume that they would be better off dead or that such burden for others is synonymous with the license to neglect or forsake that patient's essential, functional, and social best interests. Still, as Voigtlander noted, depending on the severity of the infant's retardation, the presence of further gross handicaps, or the inability of society to assist strained parents with the care of a Trisomy 21 child, one might in some extreme cases judge further treatment optional.

The concluding section of this volume will recommend a nontreatment approach hovering between that espoused by the "more restrictive" and the "broader" interpreters of the projected quality of the patient's life standard. While preserving unmitigated respect for the inherent dignity and right to life of every human patient, and related prima facie prescriptions, it still allows one to incorporate functional potential and social burden into decisions regarding the morality of foregoing treatment. Viewing each handicapped newborn as a multi-faceted rights-bearing person, parents and physicians can factor familial burden and societal limitations into a benefit/burden calculus from the patient's perspective. Such a patient bias or a weighting of the calculus on the side of the individual serves as a prudential wall against the potential abuse and selfishness on the part of burdened others that might take hold if a socially-weighted benefit/burden calculus, particularly with a functional anthropology, were allowed free reign.

NOTES

¹H. Tristam Engelhardt, Jr., "Ethical Issues in Aiding the Death of Young Children," in **Beneficent Euthanasia,** ed. Marvin Kohl, p. 18; same article also in **Killing and Letting Die,** ed. Bonnie Steinbock (Engelwood Cliffs: Prentice-Hall, 1980), p. 85.

²Carson Strong, **A Theory of Informed Consent and Proxy Consent** (Ann Arbor: University Microfilm, 1978); Strong, "Informed Consent: Theory and Policy," **Journal of Medical Ethics** 5 (December 1979), pp. 196–199; Strong, "Euthanasia: Is the Concept Really Nonevaluative?" **Journal of Medicine and Philosophy** 5 (December 1980), pp. 313–325; Strong, "Can Fluids and Electrolytes be 'Extraordinary' Treatment?" **Journal of Medical Ethics** 7 (June 1981), pp. 83–85; Strong, "Positive Killing and the Irreversibly Unconscious Patient," **Bioethics Quarterly** 3 (Fall/Winter 1981), pp. 190–205; Strong, "The Tiniest Newborns: Aggressive Treatment or Conservative Care?" **Hastings Center Report** 13 (February 1983), pp. 14–19; Strong, "Unjustified AID for the Poor?" [letter] **Hastings Center Report** 13 (August 1983), p. 50; Strong, "Defective Infants and Their Impact on Families: Ethical and Legal Considerations," **Law, Medicine and Health** 11 (September 1983), pp. 168–172; Strong [letter], **Law, Medicine and Health Care** 11 (October 1983), p. 237; Strong, "The Neonatologist's Duty to Patient and Parents," **Hastings Center Report** 14 (August 1984), pp. 10–16.

³Strong, "The Neonatologist's Duty," p. 13, parallels on pp. 14–15.

⁴Ibid., pp. 10, 13–16.

⁵Strong, "The Tiniest Newborns," pp. 14–19.

⁶Ibid., p. 16. Strong's use of percentages here is somewhat

confusing, perhaps even contradictory. On the same page he also states that "the percentage of infants with birth weights of 500–1,000 grams who survive with normal neurological outcomes varies from 5.6 percent to 29.1 percent," which seems to contradict the 45% to 78.1% statistic just noted. In either case, Strong believes that from a purely patient-centered medical standpoint aggressive treatment is warranted.

[7]C. S. Phibbs, R. L. Williams, and R. H. Phibbs, "Newborn Risk Factors and Costs of Neonatal Intensive Care," **Pediatrics** 68 (September 1981), pp. 313ff.

[8]P. Budetti, et al., "The Cost and Effectiveness of Neonatal Intensive Care," Office of Technology Assessment Background Paper #2: **Case Studies of Medical Technologies** (August 1981).

[9]A few possible sources for a fuller treatment of medical costs are Victor R. Fuchs, **Who Shall Live? Health Economics and Social Choice** (New York: Basic Books, 1974); Philip B. Heymann and Sara Holtz, "The Severely Defective Newborn: The Dilemma and the Decision Process," in **Decision Making and the Defective Newborn,** ed. Chester A. Swinyard, pp. 381–416; Marcia J. Kramer, "Ethical Issues in Neonatal Intensive Care: An Economic Perspective," in **Ethics of Newborn Intensive Care,** eds. Jonsen and Garland, pp. 75–93; John T. McCarthy, et al., "Who Pays the Bills . . . " **Journal of Pediatrics** 95 (November 1979), pp. 755–761; Office of Technology Assessment, **The Implications of Cost-Effectiveness Analysis of Medical Technology** (Washington, D.C.: U.S. Government Printing Office, August 1981).

[10]Some resources dealing with the emotional impact of a handicapped child on family and society include John Fletcher, "Attitudes Toward Defective Newborns," **Hasting Center Studies** 2 (January 1974), pp. 21–32; A. Bentovim, "Emotional Dis-

turbances of Handicapped Pre-School Children and Their Families—Attitudes to the Child," **British Medical Journal** 2 (1972), pp. 579–581; D. Drotar et al., "The Adaptation of Parents to the Birth of an Infant with a Congenital Malformation: A Hypothetical Model," **Pediatrics** 56 (1975), pp. 710ff; J. Holroyd and D. Guthrie, "Stress in Families of Children with Neuromuscular Disease," **Journal of Clinical Psychology** 35 (1979), pp. 734ff; Simon Olshansky, "Chronic Sorrow: A Response to Having a Mentally Defective Child," **Social Casework** 43 (1962), pp. 190–193.

[11]Stinson and Stinson, **The Long Dying of Baby Andrew;** Stinson and Stinson, "On the Death of a Baby," pp. 64–66 + . The Stinsons annual income of $13,600 would be taxed severely if the entire cost of Andrew's treatment ($104,403.20) fell on them. Whoever pays, was it worth it, in terms of financial costs, pain, and mental anguish? For Andrew? For others? See also: Paul Bridge and Marlys Bridge, "The Brief Life and Death of Christopher Bridge," **Hastings Center Report** 17 (December 1981).

[12]Strong, "Defective Infants and Their Impact," pp. 170, 172; Strong, "Unjustified AID for the Poor?" p. 50.

[13]Strong, "Positive Killing," pp. 193, 195–196; Strong, "Euthanasia: Is the Concept Really Nonevaluative?" p. 321. Strong's "justification can be found in the general moral principle that an action which produces a greater net good than any alternative actions in a given situation which violates no rights is morally preferable to the alternative."

[14]Bonnie Dreps Voigtlander, **An Ethical Theory for Medical Decision Making with Reference to Neonatal Intensive Care** (Ann Arbor: University Microfilms, 1979); Voigtlander, "The Role of Parents in Medical Decision Making Concerning Their Infants," in **Report of the Institute Fellows, 1977–1978,**

ed. Thomas K. McElhinney (Philadelphia: Society for Health and Human Values, 1978), pp. 303–310.

[15]Voigtlander, An Ethical Theory," p. 156, similar to p. iv.

[16]Ibid., p. 157.

[17]Ibid., p. 140.

[18]Ibid., p. 160.

[19]Ibid., p. 162.

[20]Ibid., p. 163.

[21]Ibid., p. 166.

[22]Vatican Statement, "The International Year of Disabled Persons," 747.

[23]Peter Singer, **Animal Liberation: A New Ethics for Our Treatment of Animals** (New York: Random House, 1975); Tom Regan and Peter Singer, eds., **Animal Rights and Human Obligations** (Englewood Cliffs, N.J.: Prentice-Hall, 1976); Singer, "Utility and the Survival Lottery," **Philosophy** 52 (April 1977), pp. 218–222; Singer, "Life: The Value of Life," in **Encyclopedia of Bioethics,** ed. Warren Reich, pp. 822–829; Singer, **Practical Ethics** (New York: Cambridge University Press, 1979); Singer, "Killing Humans and Killing Animals," **Inquiry** 22 (Summer 1979), pp. 145–156; Singer, "UnSanctifying Human Life," in **Ethical Issues Relating to Life and Death,** ed. John Ladd (New York: Oxford University Press, 1979), pp. 41–61; Singer and Jim Mason, **Animal Factories** (New York: Crown Publishers, 1980); Singer, "Utilitarianism and Vegetarianism," **Philosophy and Public Affairs** 9 (Summer 1980), pp. 325–337; Singer, "Can We Avoid Assigning Greater Value to Some Human Lives Than to Others?" in Center for Human Bioethics of Monash University,

Issues in Ethics (Adelaide, Australia: University of Adelaide, 1981), pp. 39–44; Singer, "How Do We Decide?" **Hastings Center Report** 12 (June 1982), pp. 9–11; Singer and Helga Kuhse, "The Future of Baby Doe," **New York Review of Books** 31 (March 1, 1984), pp. 17–22; Singer and Kuhse, **Should the Baby Live?** (New York: Oxford University Press, 1985).

Michael Tooley, "Abortion and Infanticide," **Philosophy and Public Affairs** 2 (Fall 1972), pp. 37–65; Tooley [Letter—Rebuttal to Critics plus Initial Revisions], **Philosophy and Public Affairs** 2 (Summer 1973), pp. 419–432; Tooley, "A Defense of Abortion and Infanticide," in **The Problem of Abortion,** ed. Joel Feinberg (Belmont, Cal.: Wadsworth Publishing, 1973), pp. 51–91: longer version of prior article; Tooley, "Infanticide: A Philosophical Perspective," in **Encyclopedia of Bioethics,** ed. Warren Reich, pp. 742–751; Tooley, "Decisions to Terminate Life and the Concept of Person," in **Ethical Issues Relating to Life and Death,** ed. John Ladd, pp. 62–93; Tooley, **Abortion and Infanticide** (New York: Oxford University Press, 1983).

[24]Singer, "Life: The Value of Life," p. 823; same idea found in Singer, "UnSanctifying Human Life," p. 49.

[25]Singer, **Animal Liberation,** p. 7; similar ideas also in Singer, "Can We Avoid Assigning Greater Value?" p. 40; Singer, "Life: The Value of Life," p. 826; Tooley, "A Defense of Abortion and Infanticide," p. 74; Tooley, "Infanticide: A Philosophical Perspective," p. 744; Tooley, "Decisions to Terminate Life," p. 67; Tooley, **Abortion and Infanticide,** p. 77.

[26]Singer, "Life: The Value of Life," p. 826.

[27]Tooley, "A Defense of Abortion and Infanticide," pp. 59–60; Tooley, "Infanticide: A Philosophical Perspective," pp. 745–746; Tooley, "Decisions to Terminate Life," pp. 89, 91.

[28]Tooley, **Abortion and Infanticide,** pp. 146, 164, 298, 359.

[29]Ibid., p. 360. Tooley's survey of the neurological research is found on pp. 359–371.

[30]Tooley, **Abortion and Infanticide,** pp. 407, 421. This is by contrast with his somewhat arbitrary assertion a decade earlier that at one week an infant might be accorded person status, allowing for legal infanticide prior to that cutoff: Michael Tooley, "A Defense of Abortion and Infanticide," p. 91.

[31]Tooley, "A Defense of Abortion and Infanticide," pp. 78–89; Tooley, "Infanticide: A Philosophical Perspective," pp. 746–748.

[32]Singer, "UnSanctifying Human Life," p. 48.

[33]Singer, "Life: The Value of Life," pp. 825–826; Singer, "UnSanctifying Human Life," pp. 46, 48–49; Singer, **Practical Ethics,** p. 97; Singer, "How Do We Decide?" p. 10; Tooley, "A Defense of Abortion and Infanticide," p. 79. Singer asserts somewhat arbitrarily that a healthy, mentally "normal" newborn achieves or assumes actual personhood about a month after birth: Singer, "Life: The Value," p. 826; Singer, **Practical Ethics,** pp. 136–137.

[34]Singer, **Practical Ethics,** pp. 132–133.

[35]Singer, "Life: The Value of Life," p. 824.

[36]Singer, **Practical Ethics,** pp. 133–134, 152.

[37]Ibid., p. 134; also see pp. 136–137.

[38]Singer, **Practical Ethics,** p. 138.

[39]Tooley, "Decisions to Terminate Life," pp. 80–81; similar to Tooley, "Infanticide: A Philosophical Perspective," p. 748. The phrase "morally neutral action" seems to be an overstatement, even within the Tooley-Singer schema. After all, Tooley

would seem to be in agreement with Singer's pro-animal assertions concerning the subpersonal 'quasi-right' of sentient creatures not to be pained frivolously or unnecessarily. If so, then
the willful destruction of newborns, while not synonymous with
killing actual persons, would still not be a "morally neutral action," since the subject is a sentient being, capable of being
abused if hurt needlessly.

[40]H. Tristam Engelhardt, Jr., "Viability, Abortion, and the
Difference Between a Fetus and an Infant," **American Journal
of Obstetrics and Gynecology** 116 (June 1, 1973), pp. 429–434;
Engelhardt, "Euthanasia and Children: The Injury of Continued
Existence," **Journal of Pediatrics** 83 (July 1973), pp. 170–171;
Engelhardt, "The Beginning of Personhood: Philosophical Con-
siderations," **Perkins School of Theology Journal** 27 (1973), pp.
20–27; Engelhardt, "The Ontology of Abortion," **Ethics** 84
(April 1974), pp. 217–234; Engelhardt, Kantian Knowledge of
Other Persons—An Exploration," **Akten des 4 Internationalen
Kant-Kongresses** (Mainz 6–10. April 1974), Teil 11.2; Engel-
hardt, "Solitude and Sociality," **Humanitas** 10 (November
1974), pp. 277–287; Engelhardt, "Bioethics and the Process of
Embodiment," **Perspectives in Biology and Medicine** 18 (Summer 1975), pp. 486–500; Engelhardt, "Ethical Issues in Aiding
the Death of Young Children," in **Beneficent Euthanasia**, ed.
Marvin Kohl, pp. 180–192; same article also in **Killing and Letting Die**, ed. Bonnie Steinbock, pp. 81–91; Engelhardt, "The
Counsels of Finitude," **Hastings Center Report** 5 (April 1975),
pp. 29–36; Engelhardt, "The Patient as Person: An Empty
Phrase?" **Texas Medicine** 71 (September 1975), pp. 1–7; Engelhardt, "On the Bounds of Freedom: From the Treatment of
Fetuses to Euthanasia," **Connecticut Medicine** 40 (January
1976), pp. 51–55; Engelhardt, "But Are They People?" **Hospital
Physician** 12 (February 1976), pp. 6–8; Engelhardt, "Individuals
and Communities, Present and Future: Towards a Morality in a

Time of Famine," **Soundings** 59 (Spring 1976), pp. 70–83; Engelhardt and Edmund L. Erde, "A My-T-Fine Way to Die," **Hospital Physician** 12 (June 1976), pp. 37–39; Engelhardt, "To Treat or Not to Treat—The Dilemma," **Grand Rounds, Heart and Lung** 7 (May-June 1978), pp. 499–504; Engelhardt, "Medicine and the Concept of Person," in **Ethical Issues in Death and Dying,** eds. Tom L. Beauchamp and Seymour Perlin (Englewood Cliffs, N.J.: Prentice-Hall, 1978), pp. 271–284; Engelhardt, "Rights and Responsibilities of Patients and Physicians," in **Medical Treatment of the Dying: Moral Issues,** eds. M. D. Bayles and D. M. High (Cambridge, Mass.: Schenkman Publishing, 1978), pp. 9–28; Engelhardt, "Rights to Health Care: A Critical Appraisal," **Journal of Medicine and Philosophy** 4 (June 1979), pp. 113–117; Engelhardt, "Tractatus Artis Bene Moriendi Vivendique: Choosing Styles of Dying and Living," in **Frontiers in Medical Ethics: Applications in a Medical Setting,** ed. Virginia Abernethy (Cambridge, Mass.: Ballinger, 1980), pp. 9–23; Engelhardt, "Personal Health Care or Preventive Care: Distributing Scarce Medical Resources," **Soundings** 63 (Fall 1980), pp. 234–256; Engelhardt, Jr., "Health Care Allocations: Responses to the Unjust, the Unfortunate, and the Undesirable," in **Justice and Health Care,** ed. Earl E. Shelp (Dordrecht: D. Reidel, 1984); Engelhardt, **The Foundations of Bioethics** (New York: Oxford University Press, 1986); Engelhardt, "Infanticide in a Post-Christian Age," in **Euthanasia and the Newborn,** R. C. McMillan and Engelhardt, eds. (Dordrecht: D. Reidel, 1987), pp. 81–86.

[41]Mary Anne Warren, "On the Moral and Legal Status of Abortion," **Monist** 57 (1973), pp. 43–61; Warren, "On the Moral and Legal Status of Abortion," expanded with Postscript on Infanticide, in **Today's Moral Problems,** ed. Richard Wasserstrom (New York: Macmillan Publishing Co., 1975), pp. 120–136; also in 2d ed. (1979), pp. 35–51—source for citations in this book;

also in Tom L. Beauchamp and LeRoy Walters, eds., **Contemporary Issues in Bioethics** (Belmont, Cal.: Wadsworth Publishing, 1978), pp. 217–228; Warren, "Do Potential People Have Moral Rights?" **Canadian Journal of Philosophy** 7 (1977), pp. 275–289.

[42]Warren, "On the Moral and Legal Status of Abortion," p. 48.

[43]Warren, "Do Potential People Have Moral Rights?" pp. 275–289.

[44]Warren, "On the Moral and Legal Status of Abortion," expanded with Postscript on Infanticide, p. 50.

[45]Engelhardt, "The Ontology of Abortion," p. 229.

[46]Ibid., p. 223.

[47]Ibid., p. 231.

[48]Engelhardt, "Medicine and the Concept of Person," p. 278. See also: Earle E. Shelp, **Born to Die?** (New York: The Free Press, 1987). Shelp echoes Type #4 closely, esp. Engelhardt.

[49]Engelhardt, "Medicine and the Concept of Person," p. 278.

[50]Engelhardt, "Bioethics and the Process of Embodiment," p. 498.

[51]Engelhardt, "Ethical Issues in Aiding the Death of Young Children," pp. 185–186; see also: John R. Brantley, "Wrongful Birth: The Emerging Status of a New Tort," **St. Mary's Law Journal** 8 (1976), pp. 140–159.

[52]Ibid., pp. 184, 186–187; Engelhardt, "Bioethics and the Process of Embodiment," pp. 498–499.

[53]Engelhardt, "On the Bounds of Freedom," pp. 52–53; Engelhardt, "Ethical Issues in Aiding the Death of Young Children," p. 183; Engelhardt, "Medicine and the Concept of Person," p. 278; Engelhardt, "Tractatus Artis Bene Moriendi Vivendique."

[54]Engelhardt, "Ethical Issues in Aiding the Death of Young Children," pp. 183–184.

[55]Engelhardt, "Medicine and the Concept of Person," p. 274; Engelhardt, "On the Bounds of Freedom," p. 51; Engelhardt, "Bioethics and the Process of Embodiment," p. 496; Engelhardt, "Health Care Allocations," p. 5; Engelhardt, "Tractatus Artis Bene Moriendi Vivendique," pp. 14–16.

[56]Engelhardt, "Ethical Issues in Aiding the Death," p. 185.

[57]Engelhardt, "Medicine and the Concept of Person," p. 276.

[58]Engelhardt, "Ethical Issues in Aiding the Death," p. 188.

[59]Joseph Fletcher, **Morals and Medicine** (Boston: Beacon Press, 1954); Fletcher, **Situation Ethics** (Philadelphia: The Westminster Press, 1966); Fletcher, "Euthanasia and Anti-Dysthanasia," in **Moral Responsibility: Situation Ethics at Work** (Philadelphia: The Westminster Press, 1967), pp. 141–160; Fletcher, "The Right to Die: A Theologian's Comment," **Atlantic Monthly** (April 1968), pp. 62–64; Fletcher, "What's In a Rule? A Situationist's View," in **Norm and Context in Christian Ethics,** eds. Gene Outka and Paul Ramsey (New York: Charles Scribner's Sons, 1968), pp. 325–350; Fletcher, "Ethical Aspects of Genetic Control: Designed Genetic Changes in Man," **New England Journal of Medicine** 285 (1971), pp. 776–783; Fletcher, "Indicators of Humanhood: A Tentative Profile of Man," **Hastings Center Report** 2 (1972), pp. 1–4; Fletcher,

"Medicine and the Nature of Man," **Science, Medicine and Man** 1 (1973), pp. 93–102; also in Robert Veatch, Willard Gaylin, and Councilman Morgan, eds., **The Teaching of Medical Ethics** (Hastings Center Conference Proceedings, 1973), pp. 47–58; reappears as Ch. 1 of **Humanhood: Essays in Biomedical Ethics**; Fletcher, "Ethics and Euthanasia," **American Journal of Nursing** 73 (April 1973), pp. 670–675; reprinted in **To Live and To Die: When, Why, and How**, ed. R. H. Williams (New York: Springer Verlag, 1973), pp. 113–122; also appeared, in expanded form, in **Death, Dying, and Euthanasia**, eds. Dennis J. Horan and David Mall, pp. 293–304; Joseph Fletcher, "The 'Right' to Live and the 'Right' to Die," **The Humanist** 34 (July/August 1974), pp. 12–15; also in **Beneficent Euthanasia**, ed. Marvin Kohl, pp. 44–53; Fletcher, "Four Indicators of Humanhood—The Enquiry Matures," **Hastings Center Report** 4 (December 1974), pp. 4–7; appears also under the title "What Is Humanhood?" **National Catholic Reporter** 11 (February 14, 1975), pp. 8–9; Fletcher, **The Ethics of Genetic Control: Ending Reproductive Roulette** (Garden City, N.Y.: Anchor Press/ Doubleday, 1974); Fletcher, "Moral Aspects of Decision-Making," in **Report of the Sixty-Fifth Ross Conference on Pediatric Research: Ethical Dilemmas in Current Obstetric and Newborn Care**, ed. Tom D. Moore (Columbus, Ohio: Ross Laboratories, 1976); Fletcher, " 'Sanctity of Life' vs. 'Quality of Life,' " **Contemporary Surgery** 11 (October 1977), pp. 46–47; Fletcher, "Infanticide and the Ethics of Loving Concern," in **Infanticide and the Value of Life**, ed. Marvin Kohl, pp. 13–22; also in Fletcher, **Humanhood: Essays in Biomedical Ethics**, pp. 140–148; Fletcher, "Pediatric Euthanasia: The Ethical Aspects of Selective Treatment of Spina Bifida," in **Decision Making and the Defective Newborn**, ed. Chester A. Swinyard, pp. 477–488; Fletcher, **Humanhood: Essays in Biomedical Ethics**, (Buffalo, N.Y.: Prometheus Books, 1979).

[60]Fletcher, **Morals and Medicine**, p. xviii.

[61]Fletcher, **Situation Ethics**, p. 115.

[62]Fletcher, "The Right to Die: A Theologian's Comment," p. 64.

[63]Ibid., p. 62–66.

[64]Fletcher, "Infanticide and the Ethics of Loving Concern," p. 17; Fletcher, "The 'Right' to Live and the 'Right' to Die," p. 15; Fletcher, **Humanhood: Essays in Biomedical Ethics**, p. 3.

[65]Fletcher, "Indicators of Humanhood"; Fletcher, "Medicine and the Nature of Man"; Fletcher, "Four Indicators of Humanhood"; Fletcher, "What is Humanhood?"; Fletcher, **Humanhood: Essays in Biomedical Ethics**.

[66]Fletcher, "Four Indicators of Humanhood," p. 6; Fletcher, "Ethics and Euthanasia," pp. 671–672.

[67]Fletcher, "Pediatric Euthanasia," pp. 480–481.

[68]Fletcher, "Infanticide and the Ethics of Loving Concern," p. 18.

[69]Fletcher, "Pediatric Euthanasia," p. 481.

[70]Ibid., p. 482. Paralleling Lorber's spina bifida criteria, Fletcher suggests that ambulation, mental state, urinary and fecal continence, "schoolability," and renal function might all be valid factors for the quality of the patient's life calculus (p. 483).

[71]Ibid., p. 486.

[72]Fletcher, **The Ethics of Genetic Control** (1974), p. 156.

[73]In earlier drafts this fourth ethical type was labeled "Social Utilitarianism with a Personhood Proviso." The ambiguity and debate surrounding the meaning and kinds of "utilitarian-

ism" led to a softening of that label to a "socially-weighted benefit/burden calculus." The so-called personhood proviso, while not essential to socially-weighting the decision making calculus, seems in the writings of the seven ethicists surveyed here to be sequentially-ordered as step one, prior to the application of the calculus.

[74]Gary M. Atkinson, "Persons in the Whole Sense," **American Journal of Jurisprudence** 22 (1977), pp. 86–117, esp. pp. 92–93, 111–112.

[75]Stanley Hauerwas, "Children, Suffering and the Skill to Care," pp. 147–202: Hauerwas' "ethics of care," particularly regarding the mentally handicapped, builds on this premise of "communal responsibility for" as distinguished from the "subject's obligations to" the commonweal.

[76]For a fuller treatment of the "inherent dignity" principle see the opening sections of Chapters One, Two, and Three.

[77]Philip Devine, "Nonhumans, Robots, and Infants—Infanticide and Our Industries," in **The Ethics of Homicide** (Ithaca: Cornell University Press, 1978), pp. 60–73.

[78]Tooley, "Abortion and Infanticide," p. 49; Abernethy, **Frontiers in Medical Ethics,** Introduction and pp. 3, 9, 13–14.

[79]Singer, **Practical Ethics,** p. 421.

[80]Strong, "Positive Killing," pp. 193, 195–196; Strong, "Euthanasia: Is the Concept Really Nonevaluative?" p. 321.

[81]Strong, **A Theory of Informed Consent and Proxy Consent,** esp. pp. 160–172, 184–185, 194.

[82]Voigtlander, **An Ethical Theory,** p. 140.

[83]Engelhardt, "Ethical Issues in Aiding," p. 184.

[84]**Washington Post** (December 16, 1984), interesting fact, no source or author cited.

[85]Lecture by Dr. Kenneth Rosenbaum, Director, Genetics Department, Children's Hospital National Medical Center, Washington, D.C., 14 December 1984.

[86]Russell Watson et al., "An African Nightmare," **Newsweek** (November 26, 1984): 50–55; see also Otto Friedrich, "One Miracle, Many Doubts," **Time** (December 10, 1984), pp. 70, 72; Matt Clark et al., "A Breakthrough Transplant?" **Newsweek** 12 (November 1984), pp. 114–118; Claudia Wallis, "Baby Fae Stuns the World," Time (November 12, 1984), pp. 70–72; Claudia Wallis, "Baby Fae Loses Her Battle," **Time** (November 26, 1984), pp. 88–89; Harold P. Green, "An N.I.H. Panel's Early Warnings," **Hastings Center Report** (October 1984), p. 13. Related to this is the question of massive expenditures poured into "heroic" experimental procedures for the few, which might more efficaciously be spent on the less tragically afflicted with better prognoses for life.

[87]"The Hippocratic Oath," in **Encyclopedia of Bioethics** (New York: The Free Press, 1978), p. 1731.

[88]Paul R. Johnson, "Selective Nontreatment and Spina Bifida," p. 95. Even in those macro-allocation cases, in which I tend to accept a socially-weighted calculus, it could be argued that a particular patient, as a member of the social order, "ought" to want to sacrifice narrow self-interest for the common good. Such self-sacrifice could rightly be deemed in that patient's "widest" best interest in terms of personal integrity, social responsibility, or spiritual destiny.

[89]Singer, **Practical Ethics**, pp. 78–84.

[90]Fletcher, "The Right to Die: A Theologian's Comment," p. 63.

Chapter Five

Conclusions

The concluding chapter of a survey volume can follow one of two patterns. On the one hand, it may be the denouement, the ultimate pulling together of the disparate elements that have been meticulously constructed and argued from page one right through to the now essential synthetic conclusions. Without such a concluding chapter the reader is left hanging, as if reading a mystery novel minus the final "who done it" pages. On the other hand, a survey may also be more of an analytical exposition, a thorough presentation and critique of a wide range of positions. Such a volume is usually built around a typology of some sort, with each chapter serving as a more or less self-contained unit, an explication and analysis of one of the "types" on the spectrum. Books such as H. Richard Niebuhr's **Christ and Culture** and Avery Dulles' **Models of the Church** follow this second pattern.[1] The concluding section of such a study is less essential to the integrity of the work as a whole. In Niebuhr's words, it serves largely as "a concluding unscientific postscript," an attempt to answer the nagging question: "And, finally, what do **you** think?" Of the models or types presented synthetically and systematically, where does the author stand?

The Author's Own Position
(In Light of the Typology Presented)

Between the two poles of absolute vitalism and unrestricted, libertarian autonomy lie the four ethical "types" which comprise the bulk of this volume. The medical indications or medical feasibility policy, a cousin to vitalism, rests on some commendable premises and thoughtful cautions. Whether grounded in specific Judaeo-Christian beliefs about human creation and redemption or in some natural law intuition about the human species, medical indications policy advocates espouse both the inherent personal dignity and the essential equality of every live-born human being, irrespective of functional potential or social utility. "Sanctity of Life" is an apt phrase for this presumed status and for the primacy given to the patient and his/her life preservation in medico-moral decisions. So also, medical indications proponents rightly defend a newborn patient's right to impose on family and society to sustain and nurture one's health and holistic well-being. The "canons of loyalty" between parents and offspring, health care professionals and patients, as well as the State and its citizens, mandate such stewardship duties.

Grounded in these commendable fundamental presuppositions, medical indications proponents view the signs of the times with a great deal of skepticism. The ready availability of abortion on demand, the greater societal acceptance of "death by choice" (suicide, euthanasia), and the increase in pre-natal genetic testing for the purpose of fetal abortion make Paul Ramsey and his medical indications associates ill at ease about the potential for abuse if the criteria for neonatal nontreatment follow suit. Their cautions and slippery slope fears deserve to be heard and pondered carefully by all those advocating selective nontreatment for other than reasons of medical futility.

However, mandating life-saving or life-sustaining efforts on every newborn, except those imminently and irreversibly dying or those whose conditions defy treatment, arguably constitutes "over-treatment" for some few non-dying patients, whose total well-being would thereby be subordinated to a presumption that prolonged vital signs necessarily constitute one's best interest. Ramsey's "curious exceptions" lend credence to this assertion that for some few borderline salvageable patients (the intractably pained or the permanently non-conscious) life prolongation may not be in their psychological, social, and spiritual best interests, even if physiologically feasible. Further, it seems that despite their protests to the contrary, even medical indications proponents exempt imminently dying patients from the mandatory use of interim therapies or life-sustaining devices based on **quality of** (dying) **life** or transbiological factors, not solely on some technical determination of medical benefit or "imminently dying" status as such.

Herein lies the seeds of the so-called "Sanctity of Life" versus "Quality of Life" debate that absorbed so much space in each of the first three chapters. If there is any conclusion to be drawn from the critique of Reich and Weber and the analysis of the premises of McCormick, Paris, Arras, et al., it is that for all non-vitalists these two emphases, "Sanctity of Life" and "Quality of Life," are correlated, never categorically opposed. The presumed opposition of the two, on this particular question, is a phantom dichotomy of sorts. To defend a treatment calculus in which actual or potential "burden" is ever allowed to over-ride expected medical "benefit" (life-prolongation) is to adopt some version of a results-oriented, "quality of life" ethic. It should be noted from the outset that even a patient who is reduced to "brain stem"-supported life (vital functions alone) is to be respected, accorded the "dignity" due his/her inherent, still abiding humanity or personhood. However, despite such a patient's inherent, personal dignity, one may opt to forego further life-prolongation, not as an affront to the sanctity of one's life, but as a "quality of life"-based interpretation of that patient's total best interest.

Contemporary proponents of the ordinary/extraordinary means distinction admit as much, despite their initial reluctance to allow "quality of life" language to be used. If the proposed means "cause," "are directly associated with," or even "perpetuate" a quality of the infant's life judged excessively burdensome in proportion to the expected amount of benefit, such means are declared situationally extraordinary and optional. The "means related" proviso serves as an understandable attempt to hem in these "quality of life" determinations lest the slippery slope to bias against the handicapped ensue. Linking nontreatment to the use of proposed means is another way of saying that the question we are dealing with is treatment versus nontreatment. Whether implying that an excessively burdened life, which is merely perpetuated by proposed "neutral" treatment, is in any sense a genuinely "means related" burden is questionable. "Means relatedness" seems to have been stretched beyond its logical capacities. As a restatement that we are initially dealing with the question of treatment versus nontreatment it seems redundant. It gives a false sense of objective clarity, as if the judgments are necessarily about the ordinariness or extraordinariness of **means,** rather than about the ordinary or extraordinary **quality** or condition of particular patients' lives, whether compounded by or neutrally left unchanged by proposed means.

However, contemporary ordinary/extraordinary means proponents continue to hold to the "means related" restriction in an effort to reinforce and buoy up the direct/indirect distinction and their absolute prohibition of direct infanticide, by direct acts of killing or indirectly by death-intending choices for nontreatment. Respectful of many of their fears concerning direct euthanasia, I do not see that an ambiguous denial of the quality of life basis on which the decision is made and a somewhat artificial emphasis on and stretching of "means causation" is the best way to stem the advances of the pro-euthanasia movement. Far better to acknowledge that the traditional ordinary/extraordinary means distinction is de facto a projected quality of the patient's life standard (aka Reich) and then proceed to the euthanasia question on its own turf. Whether an absolute prohibition against all direct killing of innocent patients is ethically sound or whether some leeway for a few borderline "curious exceptions" ought to be sanctioned is the stuff for a subsequent study and debate. Ramsey's curious exceptions to care, Curran's openness to direct euthanasia of some imminently dying patients, and Cahill's articulation of a Totality-based, proportionalist defense of some few acts of direct euthanasia would be recommended starting points for such a heated debate.

On the level of nontreatment questions, some contemporary proponents of the ordinary/extraordinary means distinction, namely Reich and Weber, differ very little from the more restrictive defenders of a projected quality of the patient's life standard. Both are patient-centered. Both adopt the principle of Totality, whereby excessive burden to one's holistic best interests can hold sway over potential bodily benefit. If a patient is irreversibly dying one may opt to forego interim therapies or life-sustaining devices in the name of a less burdened, more humane quality of life while dying. If the proposed means cause or contribute significantly to a quality of life during or post-treatment that is judged disproportionately burdensome **to the patient** for the degree of holistic benefit achievable, such means are optional. Whether one chooses to call the non-obligatory means "extraordinary" given the patient's life situation or to label the patient's treatment-related quality of life itself "extraordinary" is more a semantic than a substantive debate. Finally, if the patient's condition or quality of life, irrespective of means causation, is already deemed **either** so devoid of consciousness or relational potential as to derive no appreciable benefit from life-sustaining treatment **or else,** even if minimally relational, is inordinately burdened by pain, suffering, or grave inconvenience, then all therapeutic and life-sustaining treatments are arguably not in the patient's best interest. They become optional, regardless of their life-saving and death-forestalling capability.

Concerning the question of the incorporation of "burden to others" into the nontreatment calculus, contemporary ordinary/extraordinary means proponents seem more reluctant than the antecedent ordinary/extraordinary means tradition to stretch the interpretation of the patient's best interests so wide. In the same way, those projected quality of the patient's life advocates labeled "more restrictive" either categorically exclude social burden factors in the cases of non-competent patients (Veatch, Arras) or else exclude the legitimacy of familial burden and then decline to comment further on wider societal burden and resource limitations (McCormick, Paris). In both nontreatment approaches the determination of burden for the handicapped newborn patient seems to be restricted almost exclusively to individualistic patient-experienced pain, suffering, and inconvenience. The exorbitant "costs" of prolonged care, which traditionally were incorporated as a burden factor, seem to be invalid content in the cases of newborns, simply because others pay the bills. Ought not the financial and emotional limits of these "others" be factored in as part of the burden incurred by this socially-contexted patient?

It seems that both the means-related ordinary/extraordinary means proponents and the more restrictive quality of the patient's life advocates too readily assume that inexhaustible resources exist or that Pius XII's "grave burden to oneself **or another**" [my emphasis] is not applicable in the cases of newborns and other non-competents. Provided one takes rightful and respectful caution against too facile a refusal of treatment for an infant based on minimal familial or societal "costs," it seems fair to incorporate the financial and emotional costs associated with one's treatment, at least as a correlative factor in computing net burden related to the patient's own well-being.

The broader interpreters of the projected quality of the patient's life approach do in fact push the boundary of burden-to-the-patient to its rightful wider limits by incorporating social concerns as one element in determining a given patient's net best interest. While this author is ill at ease with and critical of the heavily bourgeois, normalcy-biased value system operative in the case applications discussed by Duff, Campbell, and Lorber, that does not mean that Shaw's "H" and "S" factors, burden to one's family and society, should categorically be excluded from the patient's best interest calculus. At least with reference to competent patients, burden to one's social milieu has been an admissible element in the nontreatment calculus of ordinary/extraordinary means tradition, provided social factors are seen as they impact on the patient's own objective and experiential best interests, not as factors stacked over against the patient. Hellegers' example of a husband opting to forego seriously debilitating brain surgery at least partly because of his personal desire not to overburden his loved ones is a paradigmatic illustration. In a very real sense, the thought of heavily burdening his family adds a significant burden to his own benefit/burden calculus, potentially tipping the scales in favor of nontreatment.

The subsequent question seems to be whether such social burden can or ought to be filtered into the benefit/burden calculus concerning a newborn's best interests. A similar question would be raised in the case of any non-competent patient for whom no prior wishes, value system, or sense of commitment to family/society can be discerned. Can we presume that a handicapped newborn patient with a physiologically-related quality of life judged **either** totally devoid of experiential relational potential **or** else quite burdened, but not necessarily excessively so, would factor in his/her burdensomeness to parents and others, possibly tilting the scale from seeing one's own life as minimally worth preserving to "extraordinarily burdened"? Can we impute societal responsibility to a patient who is presently incapable of guilt or culpability for the strain one is objectively causing one's significant others?

An argument can be made analogous to one set forth by Gilbert Meilaender against Ramsey's medical indications tendency to deny to non-competent patients the right to factor individualized "burden" elements into decisions for/against treatment, a right he seemingly grants to competent adults. As Meilaender summarized it, a medical indications policy "seems to leave us in the unhappy position of making imperative for infants treatments which many competent patients would decline for themselves—accepting for all infants what only some or, perhaps few of the rest of us might accept for ourselves."[2] The parallel with the incorporation of social burdens seems obvious. To allow competent adults the license to factor in familial burden, which the ordinary/extraordinary means and quality of the patient's life proponents readily admit, while at the same time excluding such a right to non-competents, as exercised by their entrusted proxies or guardians, seems to be a species of bias against them, however well intended. Phrased more positively, if "grave burden to another" is an appropriate element in the calculus to determine what constitutes excessive burden for a competent patient, it ought also to be apropos for infants and other non-competents, provided their substituted decision makers exercise extreme caution to avoid conflicts of interest. Potential abuse may call for adequate checks and balances, perhaps in the form of Infant Care Review Committees or court hearings prior to cessation of treatment in those cases where social factors are involved, not a categorical exclusion of familial burden as valid input.

Such a schema, in which social burden factors enter into judgments concerning a neonatal patient's holistic quality of life, applies to decisions for and against treatment as follows. If a newborn patient is irreversibly dying, one generally ought to choose the course of interim therapy or nontreatment that will facilitate the best quality of life for that now dying patient. If proposed interim therapies are judged medically futile or inordinately wasteful, it might be argued that further use becomes not merely "optional," but actually "contra-indicated." If a seriously handicapped newborn is not irretrievably dying, but if s/he has a course of treatment to look forward to that in itself is judged **excessively** painful and inconvenient **for that infant**, such a series is optional. So also, if the infant's functional potential is so devoid of "experience-ability" or one's handicapped condition is itself extraordinarily burdensome, then future therapeutic treatments, even for relatively unrelated illnesses, seem practically useless and are not obligatory.

All of these precede and in some sense prescind from social factors. However, if a **severely** handicapped non-dying infant, especially one with barely any or no "conscious" relational potential, faces a course of treatment that is not necessarily inordinately painful in itself, but which will totally bankrupt one's family and/or contribute to a parent's probable mental breakdown and/or deprive a number of other needy patients with far better prognoses of life-saving medical resources, it is possible that that patient's **total** best interests—including psychological, social, and spiritual well-being—might be better served by nontreatment. Continued minimal life experience for the patient at such a high cost to one's primary caretakers or to one's fellow NICU residents in some instances may constitute too much burden for too little medical and experiential benefit. I am not proposing a socially-weighted calculus, in which the best interests of a newborn with a reasonably good prognosis can be over-ridden by social factors, but rather a patient-centered calculus, in which social factors may compound an already negative prognosis. See the case application section (the Case of Betsy Novick) for a possible scenario of this type.

No doubt the incorporation of such "H" and possibly "S" factors would have to be done cautiously, aware that others may want to cease the good fight too soon for selfish motives. It might even be argued that such an ethically permissible schema ought to be outlawed in public policy solely to forestall utilitarian abuse. Still, the ordinary/extraordinary means tradition, as expressed by Pius XII, and the broader interpreters of the quality of the patient's life approach are correct to defend that in ethical discourse one's social impact ought not categorically be excluded in calculating burden and benefit in one's holistic best interests.

The writings of D'Youville College professor Paul R. Johnson serve as the best articulation of this mid-course between a projected quality of the patient's life standard so restrictive as to be almost exclusively based on physiological capacities and individualist burden determinations and one so broad that it too readily allows usually bearable familial burden to over-ride a functionally able infant's individual interest in life-saving therapy.[3] Referring to Shaw's quasi-mathematical formula, Johnson says that some amalgam of biological deficiencies and burden, coupled with familial inadequacies, and finally compounded by limited societal health care resources, may indicate in some instances that the best or even only option is nontreatment. He goes on to suggest that factoring in social concerns may also, at times, tilt the scale in the opposite direction, **toward** treatment, especially where a society is solvent enough to back its pro-life preference with sufficient health care and life-enhancing resources. He notes that a general policy of aggressive life support for newborns serves as a symbolic statement to society, assuring all of us that we will never be abandoned, even if feeble or defenseless. However, he cautions care lest these seeming best interest concerns be turned into vitalistic mandates for **our** peace of mind against a particularly burdened patient's own best interest in ceasing treatment.

Conclusions

Johnson commends the government of this country both for Public Law 94-142 and for Section 504 of the Rehabilitation Act (Public Law 93-112), each of which mandates societal responsibility and funding for the care and further life support of handicapped persons destined for treatment. Generally speaking, if the financial or psychic cost of a handicapped child's care overtaxes one's family, the society should accept the child into its social service purview as an instance of **parens patriae** responsibility. Still, one need not always mandate treatment, irrespective of a society's finite limitations. For example, if a given infant were to require an artificial heart, permanent dialysis or a kidney transplant, plus a "bubble" environment to substitute for one's deficient immune system, society might from the outset say "no," either in terms of a socially-weighted macro-allocation calculus concerning equitable distribution of limited resources, or, as Johnson would prefer, in terms of the patient's best interest, socially as well as individualistically considered. This author echoes Johnson both in acknowledging the potential for patient abuse if social factors are not monitored carefully and in refusing to categorically outlaw social burden as one more ethically valid factor in determining an infant patient's wider best interest.

Finally, this possibility that society, in some instances, might say "no" to a patient's valid individualistic interest in treatment brings us face to face with Type Four, a socially-weighted benefit/burden calculus, in which the interests and rights of handicapped newborns no longer are absolute, but instead can be outweighed by other interests and concerns. The authors gathered at this end of the spectrum deserve some degree of credit for their strong, though **overstated** articulation of two points:

(1) for challenging any definition of the patient's well-being that hinges treatment/nontreatment so completely on in-

herent personhood and the presumption toward prolongation of life in its physiological aspects that one's quality
of life or functional potential becomes a non-factor;

(2) for incorporating social concerns, which, in turn, raise
valid questions concerning scarce or finite resources and
the limits this inevitably places on any patient's access to
unlimited treatment.

1. Regarding the first of these two points, I believe that in
sweeping out the demon of a physiology-biased definition of patient's best interest and a correlative vitalistic approach to nontreatment decisions, proponents of a socially-weighted benefit/
burden calculus have swept in a **far greater** anthropological demon. In order to incorporate factors related to the patient's psychological, social, and spiritual potential, one need not **and
ought not** negate that patient's fundamental or inherent worth
as a human person.

In contrast to this approach I have proposed a multi-leveled
interpretation of the patient's well-being or personal best interest, which builds upon the affirmed premise that live-born membership in the human species is **sufficient** ground to declare
every human being a person, inherently valuable and rights-
laden. While being a person, in the sense of being physically
alive, is a sufficient basis on which to generally mandate life-prolongation as presumably in a given patient's best interest, his/her
actual best interest or well-being is much broader and ought to
incorporate more elements or human goods. One way of phras-
ing this is to say that one has "life" or is alive, in the physiological
sense, for other purposes, to foster and further one's holistic best
interests. On the psychological or rational level, one's best interests may be construed in terms of mental or upper brain development. On a social level, it may be construed in terms of
one's ability, however minimally, to ingest, process, and respond
to relational input. From a spiritual or theological perspective,

one's life is oriented toward fulfillment in God—reflected in a faith relationship here and in eternal transcendent union hereafter.

Therefore, the total destruction or absence of one's embodied capacities for experiential participation in the psychological, social, and penultimate spiritual aspects of one's dynamic well-being would indicate a patient whose embodiment is already seriously deficient and/or substantially extinguished and whose continued need for and use of the remaining physiological aspects of life (i.e., basic vital signs) is proportionately less. If one's physiological life is so maimed or reduced as to offer one very little or no possibility for further embodied psychological, social, or earthly spiritual flourishing (i.e., one's upper brain is dead or practically so or so absorbed in suffering), then the usually beneficial and morally mandatory prolongation of the basic physiological aspects of one's life ceases to be compelling. Without rejecting one's respiration or circulation in any direct way, and without denying one's abiding, inherent dignity, one may morally opt for nontreatment in the name of the patient's wider best interests.

If one has the functional potential both for psychological activity and relational interaction, even on a fairly primitive level, then one's life can be said to be "meaningful" to the patient. Barring excessive burden for the patient (including familial and social concerns), and barring a categorical absence of health care resources, such patients ought to be treated. If, on the other hand, one even lacks such minimal potential, then one's capacity for embodied human flourishing can be said to have ended (not merely "reached its potential," as McCormick suggests). Barring any reason, arising from particular social circumstances, for prolonging such a patient's life, no further life-saving or life-sustaining treatment seems warranted **in that patient's best interest,** holistically-viewed.

Using Burghardt's threefold metaphor, "sheer life" is a

symbol of one's abiding intrinsic worth as a human person. If there is no embodied, brain-related potential for "good life," one's experiential participation in the goods of human flourishing, then "sheer life" loses its actual significance or value **to the patient** so suspended between mere existence and "eternal life." Life-saving or merely life-sustaining medical efforts become situationally futile. Nontreatment, with a legitimate desire that death may come sooner, becomes the most life-respecting option.

2. The second valid issue raised by the socially-weighted benefit/burden "type" is that burden to others, in terms of financial and emotional costs, ought not categorically be excluded from the treatment/nontreatment calculus. Acknowledging social factors leads one to important questions related to the distribution of finite resources. Sometimes the valid needs and limited capacities of others (the Common Good) or even society's triage interest in saving "X" instead of "Y" may understandably compete with a given patient's **individualistic** interest in treatment. Ultimately, proponents of each type made allowance for some kind of a social calculus in extreme, perhaps only hypothetical cases. Surely one's analysis of world resources, budgetary priorities, and whether there is a real resource crisis will color one's inclusion or general exclusion of such macro-allocation issues.

The data is far too complex and the questions too hotly debated to be accurately and adequately summarized here. Still, a few "thought starters" might be raised in question form. Given the gross material and financial inequities between the first and third world cultures, does the amount of money and talent invested in cutting edge medical technology and cures (e.g., Neonatology) in the industrialized North and West constitute an injustice toward the rightful health care needs of persons in the Southern or Eastern hemispheres? Within one's own national or regional culture, what percentage of our finite resources should be invested in health care as opposed to nutrition, housing, education, safety, defense, the arts, and other human needs? Within the health care budget itself, how much should go to therapeutic medicine versus research? To adults versus children? To the most curable versus the chronically ill? To the elderly versus the young? To those who can pay versus to those in need but without funds? All of these are valid and interrelated questions which, to some extent, nuance and counterbalance any handicapped newborn's best interest, if defined in psychological, social, and spiritual as well as physiological terms.[4] Carson Strong and the other proponents of a socially-weighted benefit/ burden calculus raise these questions and refuse to simply assume that "cost effectiveness" is a non-issue in decisions regarding severely handicapped infants with prognoses for exorbitantly costly, perhaps only minimally beneficial courses of treatment.

However, I have rejected the adoption of a socially-weighted calculus as the solution to these valid social concerns within the case-by-case practice of medical decision making. It flies in the face of the Hippocratic tradition, which sees the physician, within his/her practice of medicine, solely as the patient's advocate, one who comes "for the benefit of the sick."[5] Contrary to Strong's assertion, the parents are not the doctor's clients. Their interests, while valid, ought to remain secondary to the patient's, incorporated in a subsidiary capacity only as they impact on the infant's totality. So also, the parents and physician are not delegates of the State, if by that one implies some socialistic obligation on their part to conserve society's resources over against the infant-patient's needs. Rather, if parents and physicians serve in any delegated capacity at all, it is as responsible guardians, caretakers entrusted with the best interests of voiceless offspring/patients. The "art" of medicine, including ethical decision making, is and ought to remain a patient-centered venture.

Therefore, assuming some validity to these **questions re-**

lated to finite health care resources, and yet extremely reluctant to adopt a social utilitarian approach to actual treatment decision making, I recommend two methodological options, each of which would allow for resource limitations without denigrating a patient's worth or underestimating his/her claim to available resources:

(1) One can openly adopt a socially-weighted, "Common Good"-oriented calculus on the global/national/regional macro-allocation level, making prior and categorical determinations concerning budgetary priorities. Based on these pre-case, pre-cribside determinations, certain genera or species of cases will be a priori excluded as too costly, too futile, or too inequitable a distribution of regrettably finite resources. From that point on, all intra-system medical decisions for or against treatment ought to be patient-centered, based solely on the patient's holistic best interest. Thus, an absolute line of demarcation is drawn between inevitable budgetary limitations set on health care resources, which exclude some expenditures as fundamentally socially un-just, and medico-moral decision making itself, which has tradi-tionally been centered exclusively on the patient and should continue to be so focused.

(2) The second option is to stretch the concept of best in-terest not only to include familial burden, but one's social re-sponsibilities as well. In such a schema, exorbitant costs for a course of treatment deemed wasteful, given a severely retarded, intractably pained, or permanently non-conscious infant's rela-tive lack of potential for benefit, would make such treatment op-tional with the assumption that such a patient, if competent, could, and perhaps even "should," opt not to overtax his/her community for "futile" life-prolongation. Such a broadened interpretation of the patient's best interest would seem most helpful in the cases of permanently non-conscious non-dying pa-tients, for whom extraordinary burden to self is difficult to dem-onstrate if restricted solely to that individual's conscious

experience of burden. Seeing societal as well as familial burden as valid though subsidiary elements of a patient's personal best interest allows all nontreatment decisions, even those dealing with macro-allocation issues, to be patient-centered.

"Let's Get Down to Cases"

In the final analysis no methodological approach or list of ethical criteria passes moral muster unless it works in actual case applications. There is general agreement to exempt anencephalic babies from further life-sustaining efforts and a quasi-absolute mandate that Down's Syndrome infants with digestive blockages should be treated, barring unforeseen complicating factors. What about the broad spectrum in between? Who, according to the synthetic type just espoused, should be treated or not treated?

Four cautions or procedural perimeters need to be stated up-front.

(1) As McCarthy, Jonsen, Garland, and others have forcefully argued, there should be no rush to judgment. Suggesting that "time is a commodity we usually have," pediatric intensivist Murray Pollack cautions against precipitous decision making in the neonatal or early infancy period.[6] Accurate diagnoses and prognoses for physiological and functional potential frequently require further testing, observation, and time to become "mature" or reasonably "certain." When in doubt, wait and see. Presume on the side of life-prolongation.

(2) Beware of the "technical criteria fallacy."[7] Whatever list of congenital anomalies, prenatal or neonatal traumas, and diseases one projects as lethal, painful, or constituting poor prognoses, the ethical decision for or against treatment is broader. It does not rest solely or wholly on these physiological indicators. Even in those instances where such factors (e.g., medical futility) rule the calculus, the other components are at least theoretically

valid. In other cases, the transbiological elements of suffering, cost, inconvenience, and social burden may even override the medical benefit of life-prolongation itself, if treatment were to be accepted.

(3) Related to this is a concern expressed earlier against the ordinary/extraordinary means tradition for giving the impression that one can declare species of means universally "ordinary" or "extraordinary." Such relative or generic categorizations need to be posited with humble tentativeness. To imply that the illustrative case scenarios which follow are in any sense absolute is to offer a false impression of ethical objectivity. Given the subjective element of parental and physician intentionality and the unique twists of medical and circumstantial factors and assessments, the case applications listed here are projected "maybes," possible instances in which, all things being equal, nontreatment ought to be an option.

(4) It should be noted that parents, health care professionals, and even handicapped survivors are frequently critical of ethicists who do not actually spend time in the NICU, experiencing at least vicariously their anguish and trauma. Such criticism, bordering at times on hostility, bespeaks a concern that the emotional intensity of parenting, medically dealing with, or actually being a severely handicapped child cannot and ought not be passed over or under-valued in ethical analyses. For every reason cited to defend the potential value of a dispassionate, objective, rational decision maker, one might counter with concern that emotional burden, subjective "cope-ability," and intuition are essential situational elements that cannot and should not be underestimated.

One can draw two conclusions from this last criticism and/ or hostility. First, an ethicist rightly ought to experience and empathize with those parents, professionals, and patients s/he is going to write about in order to realistically and humanely ground one's scholarship. In this regard, I owe a debt of gratitude to the patients, parents, and dedicated staff of Children's Hospital National Medical Center for affording me the opportunity for such an experiential component of my research. Second, the complexity, anguish, and cutting edge nature of truly "gray" or borderline decisions call for respectful sensitivity, both in decision making and in subsequent retrospective critique. Upon careful reflection neither alternative may be obviously or categorically correct. Between the generally bleak case of an anencephalic baby and the usually hopeful case of a Trisomy 21 child lies a lot of gray.

At the most obvious nontreatment end of the spectrum the anencephalic newborn is not alone. There are a number of terminal, static, practically untreatable conditions whose victims ought to be made comfortable and humanely accompanied to death's door. Exencephaly, hydranencephaly, and holoprosencephaly are some of the more common and readily detectable of these terminal, brain-related conditions. The holoprosencephalic infant has a "very dismorphic brain," in which the two halves failed to differentiate and develop compartmentally. A severely squashed face with all the features "pushed together" is the obvious symptom that such a condition exists. Hydranencephaly refers to an infant born already suffering the ravages of intrauterine hydrocephalus. Neonatal shunting may prevent the infant's head from swelling further, but is already too late to prevent **severe** fluid-related brain damage. Inside the newborn's scull remains "not even a rim of brain," but "just a piece of tissue that once was brain."[8] These infants have **no** cognitive activity or relational potential. Death is usually imminent within hours, days, or weeks. However, there is one documented case of an anencephalic child who lived until the age of ten, totally nonconscious, presumably sustained by an extraordinarily hardy brain stem. Given their total inability to participate even minimally in the goods of human flourishing as well as the obvious burden their birth and care must be for family and caretakers, such infants should not be sustained on ventilators nor given interim therapies for other relatively treatable conditions. Lacking any experiential quality of life, it is in their eternal and social best interests not to have vital signs sustained artificially nor to have penultimate life prolonged needlessly.

Several other brain-related "defects" are less easily diagnosed in the first minutes or hours after delivery, but can be confirmed as severe, untreatable, and terminal by chromosome studies or other diagnostic tests. In this category are babies born with Trisomy 13 and Trisomy 18. Can they be said to be lacking all relational potential? Here the difficulty of technical criteria and of the ambiguity of terminology come to the fore. Frequently, relational function is linked to brain activity by the term "consciousness." An ethicist's inquiry might run something like this: "Is this Trisomy 13 infant [with the collapsed face, pimento-like eye slits, and dried up grapefruit-like head] 'conscious'?" The infant's physician might respond, "Yes, she is 'conscious,' if by 'conscious' you mean what medicine means by consciousness. She does have intermittent periods of sleep and wakefulness." "No," the ethicist might respond, "I mean: Is she 'aware'?" A slight, but firm tap to the infant's foot elicits a reflex leg reaction and a weak cry, so the neonatologist responds, "If you mean 'Are her nerve endings operative and can she feel pain?' yes, she is 'aware.'" Then the medical specialist might add, "But the real question ought to be: 'Is she **responsive**?'" Included in this is the presumption of some level of interpersonal relationship, not solely pain-sensitive nerve endings. After a reasonable number of weeks of post-natal evolution will a Trisomy 13 infant begin to smile or coo or perk up upon hearing her mother's voice? Will the primary care nurse's gentle touch or cradling 'relax' her? Will the Trisomy 13 baby show facial signs of "responding" to care? The answer is "no."

In that sense a Trisomy 13 or a Trisomy 18 baby can be said to be non-relational, but surely not as blatantly so as wholly non-conscious anencephalic infants. Terminology and functional categories seem to be less definitive and less precise in actual practice than in ethical theory. Fortunately, such infants are also irretrievably dying, so that even if life-sustainers and interim therapies could offer these babies some brief opportunity for extremely doubtful levels of human affirmation, the "burdens" of treatment seem to far outweigh the "benefit" for so little experience and so short a time. Similarly, babies born cycloptic (one-eyed with seriously dismorphic brains) or with severe microencephaly or with any other major congenital brain anomaly can be said either to be irretrievably dying, or, even if not, so mentally non-cognitive as to have no experiential interest in life-sustainers or interim therapies.

The cases of newborns who have suffered **severe** pre-natal or neonatal asphyxia and those who have sustained most forms of Grade Four intra-ventricular hemorrhages also test out to be similarly non-relational, lacking all "conscious" upper brain activity. The functional prognoses for these trauma-induced brain deficiencies are less predictable immediately following birth or the post-partum incident. Various amounts of time and neurological testing are required before one can with any degree of prognostic certainty predict such a baby's cognitional future. From one perspective, these are cases in which there is no need to decide quickly. However, these may also be cases in which a child sustained on a ventilator during that prognostic interim may "recover" to a mental state below relationality or consciousness but sufficient to sustain respiration again on one's own. In such cases, the decision to wait also represents a missed opportunity for cessation of ventilator assistance. Such a child has been launched by interim respiratory therapy and the debatable benefit of time into an arguably "meaningless" or even excessively burdened life in experiential terms.

There are also a number of rare, major malformations that are not brain-related, but which nonetheless are severely burdensome, incurable, and inevitably terminal. Sirenomelia sequence (Mermaid Syndrome), which occurs only once in every 60,000 births, is an example of this kind of rare untreatable condition. The infant's mermaid-like undivided limbs are an exterior sign of interior lung, heart, and brain abnormalities. Beyond palliative care and procedures undertaken to assist patient management while dying, further life-prolongation efforts are unwarranted.[9]

Several other severe conditions—hypoplastic left or right ventricle (small underdeveloped heart), hypoplastic lungs (small, undeveloped lungs), the absence of kidneys, and necrotizing enterocolitis (dying bowel/colon)—present decision-makers with debatable prognoses and treatment options. Currently some experimental surgical and transplant procedures are being offered to some hypoplastic heart infants (e.g., Loma Linda's Baby Fae). The cutting edge, largely experimental nature of such procedures could generally be judged as too little potential benefit, at present, for the projected cost, pain, and inconvenience to the probably terminal newborn. Such procedures would seem to be optional. Likewise, the technology exists to put hypoplastic lung sufferers on **permanent** home ventilator care or to sustain a patient with necrotizing enterocolitis or a very short gut **permanently** on TPN (Total Parenteral Nutrition), at a cost of at least $30,000 to $50,000 per child, per year. However, if one is missing a vital organ or a vital organ system, it seems at least arguably excessive and inordinate to artificially substitute for that essential function on a permanent basis. The prospect of lifelong ventilator dependency or of constant TPN in these cases can be labeled extraordinary beyond one's presumed obligation to prolong and foster life. The burden associated with machine dependence, cost, and potential medical complications would, at the present time, make such treatment highly questionable and surely non-obligatory.

Thus far we have dealt with a series of birth defects or diseases in which "dying is irreversibly proximate" unless fore-stalled by life-sustainers or in which the infant's "relational potential is negligible."[10] The quality of life open to such patients is either nil or for such a short duration of time as to be optionally not worth the individual's pain and inconvenience nor the cost and strain on the newborn's family and society. Treatment is categorically burdensome for no measureable experiential benefit. The best treatment would be nontreatment, save for humane palliative, hygienic, and, where appropriate, nutritional care.

Are there cases, in which the newborn patient is not dying in any proximate sense and in which the infant is at least minimally responsive to significant others, that might still be candidates for nontreatment based on excessive burden or intractable pain or borderline inordinate burden compounded by social burden factors? The answer, according to the projected quality of the patient's life approach adopted here, would be "yes" to all three possible schemas. Illustrative case scenarios will be offered for each.

1. Excessive Burden to the Non-Dying Newborn Patient

Baby Fred, the newborn child of a severely diabetic mother, was born slightly premature, suffering from very low hemoglobin and hematic rates (related to the mother's diabetes) and an oomphalocele (bowel protruding through the umbilicus). The child became hydropic (fluids "all over" body cavity) due to the anemia, which prompted the hospital of origin to invest thirty-six hours in stabalizing therapies. During this time the infant sustained fairly severe hypoxia. Rushed to a regional NICU at this point, Baby Fred was found to have "persistent fetal circulation," a belated continuation of the in utero circulation pattern, in which blood tends to move away from, rather than toward the infant's formerly unused lungs. This condition required high pressures and oxygenation to force enough oxygen to the brain to sustain life and to forestall further brain damage.

When the child finally "woke up" he was maintained on Pavulon, a curare-like paralyzing drug, which allowed the team to artificially breathe for the infant's malfunctioning lungs.

After this, Baby Fred had a seizure, followed by a markedly abnormal, but not flat brain wave. The patient developed cardiomyopathy, a thickening and enlarging of the heart muscle, probably an undesired side-effect of the blood pressure medications. Baby Fred's prognosis for survival is bleak, but death is neither imminent nor presently irreversible. His mental ability is minimal, but not categorically non-cognitive nor relationally void. The infant's amalgam of medical problems now include:

1. a very abnormal brain wave, indicating probable severe, static retardation;

2. the oomphalocele, still requiring corrective surgery;

3. severe chronic lung disease, necessitating permanent respirator aid;

4. severe cardiac problems related to the myopathy and two small septal defects, all requiring further corrective surgeries;

5. a respiratory virus related to the continued use of high pressures;

6. catheter-related clotting in the superior and inferior **vena cava.**

Finally, while facial expression and muscle tension are not airtight indicators of a newborn's "feelings," the experienced health care team say that this baby "looks pained" and "uncomfortable." As his neonatologist states it, "the look on his face when someone touches him is anything but happy. He looks as though life is not worth the effort."

If such prognoses and observation-based interpretations

are at all accurate, continued treatment is arguably inhumane. In the best interests of Baby Fred, so burdened by his basic congenital defects, by hypoxia-induced brain damage, by the complicating anomalies caused by various essential therapies, and by the prospect of almost inevitable further medical complications as well as lifelong ventilator dependence, his parents and the health care team may well opt for a two stage course of nontreatment. First, they might declare the infant a "no code" patient, which forbids resuscitative efforts if and when the baby has a future seizure or cardiac arrest. Second, after a reasonable span of time with no physiological improvement or perhaps as Baby Fred's condition compounds itself, they might decide to remove the infant from the respirator, allowing him to die.

In this case scenario the patient's quality of life—a combination of multiple anomalies compounded by an escalating, oppressive, and largely maintenance course of treatment—can be judged extraordinarily burdensome **to the patient**. His personal, social, and spiritual interests may be served best by nontreatment (i.e., cessation of life-sustaining ventilator assistance).

2. Intractable Pain for the Infant Not "Imminently" Dying

For a case that represents or approximates intractable pain or suffering one might reread Bonnie Dreps Voigtlander's third case, summarized in Chapter Four, that of an infant with the rare genetic skin disease called dystropic epidermolysis bullosa of the recessive form.[11] Capable of surviving to the age of five or so, a baby with this disease suffers the following symptoms:

> Repeated episodes of blistering, infection and scar formation lead to severe deformities, loss of hair, buccal mucosal scarring, dysphagia, and retarded physical and sexual development . . . toe and finger lesions heal with fusions of digits and loss of nails.[12]

Even medical indications proponent Paul Ramsey exempts such a non-dying patient from further life-saving or life-sustaining efforts, though he declines to acknowledge that it is in the patient's best interests to do so, opting instead for his curious "beyond care" exception. Voigtlander reports that despite reasonable doses of demaril for palliation, the baby "screamed with pain and/or anticipation of pain" throughout the daily bath and dressing routine. Alert and developing neurologically well, such infants understandably may become suspect of bodily touch, mentally distancing themselves at least from one avenue of human inter-action. Familial frustration and stress may be added as corroborative burden factors, but not essentially or necessarily so. The quality of life open to this child is either so irremediably pained or else so doped up (relationally non-conscious) that should life-sustainers be required or treatment become necessary for pneumonia, infections, or other curable diseases, one might opt to forego these efforts in the patient's holistic best interests, hoping for ("desiring," not necessarily morally "intending") an earlier and easier rather than a belabored and painful dying process.

Based on currently available data, one is not able to declare whether Tay Sachs disease or Lesch-Nyhan syndrome, frequently mentioned in the ethical literature, rightly ought to be considered intractably pained conditions. Certainly the early months of life with either anomaly are relatively burden free. The four to five year projected lifespan for victims would generally prevent one from labeling such patients as imminently dying. Still, if excessive burden includes suffering as well as physiological pain, then a reasonable person might evaluate the later symptoms of each condition as excessively burdensome qualities of life, beyond what a child ought to be expected to bear, especially with a terminal prognosis of death before school age. In the case of Tay Sachs disease these symptoms include mental retardation, susceptibility to other diseases, convulsions, sluggishness, apathy, failure to fix objects with one's eyes, inability to take an interest in one's surroundings, loss of motor reactions, inability to sit up or to hold one's head up, loss of weight, muscle atrophy, blindness, pseudobulbar palsy, inability to feed orally, decerebrate rigidity and gross physical deformity. The tragic symptoms of Lesch-Nyhan syndrome are somewhat similar. The patient is mentally retarded, unable to walk or even to sit unassisted, and is prone to uncontrollable spasms. As noted earlier, the most traumatic symptom of Lesch-Nyhan patients of teething age is self-mutilation, their tendency to gnaw their own lips, tongue, fingers, and appendages to nubs.

Ramsey noted in passing "some small degree of success" that Dr. William Nyhan has been having in developing a drug to relieve the non-neurological symptoms of the disease which bears his name.[13] Likewise, researchers at the National Institutes of Health are embarking on an experimental study of effects of gene therapy on heretofore incurable Lesch-Nyhan sufferers. The palliative or even therapeutic results of these efforts would have to be studied before one could include or exclude Lesch-Nyhan syndrome from the short list of irremediably painful anomalies. Since physiological pain is only a subset, not the sum and substance of what constitutes human suffering, I tend to agree with Beauchamp, Childress, and Veatch that somewhere along the course of care from birth to pre-school death, these two anomalies constitute qualities of life in which the child is so caught up in the mere effort to cope with suffering that further curative treatments for other medical problems are optionally unwarranted. Death from pneumonia or sepsis at age two or three is potentially more humane and life-respecting than a slow, lingering death at age five preceded by two or three years of the symptoms listed above.

3. Patient Burden Compounded By Social Burden Factors

The case of Baby Betsy Novick serves as a possible paradigm of an infant whose basic quality of life, course of treatment, and negative social factors coalesce to constitute a life excessively burdened for too little personal benefit. At birth Betsy Novick was diagnosed as having Seckel syndrome or "bird-headed" dwarfism, an autosomal recessive genetic disease. Symptoms include low birth weight and length, large eyes, a large beaklike nose, narrow face, receding lower jaw, strabismus, a club foot, and moderately severe retardation related to the gross cerebral deformation.

The Novick family was familiar with the care problems related to Seckel syndrome since Mr. Novick's brother had also suffered its effects. "The Novicks were of modest means and the vivid memory of the devastating impact of Mr. Novick's brother immediately convinced him that the child could not be cared for at home."[14] However, they lived in a state that has the lowest per capita income spent on institutions for the mentally handicapped. Despite some court action promising marginal improvements in the state's "asylums," they still promised to be "bleak, understaffed, custodial institutions for the foreseeable future." Given the baby's fairly repugnant facial features and stunted size, her parents feared that she might be shunned by her custodial keepers and receive even less than her fair share of already sub-standard care. Still, they saw no manageable alternative.

In the next two months Betsy developed a persistent pyloric stenosis, a narrowing of the pylorus between the stomach and the intestines, which caused projectile vomiting. Drug therapy and a special diet failed to cure the condition, necessitating immediate surgery to allow for proper digestion and nutritional sustenance. The parents, initially stunned by this additional life-threatening complication, attempted to weigh the practical alternatives in Betsy's best interests. Perceiving Betsy's projected quality of life over the next decade or so in any institution available to them to be one of "severe burden and suffering," they decided that was a burden their child ought not bear, even though in principle they believed that society should be acting as **parens patriae** in Betsy's behalf. Therefore, they opted to withhold consent for the surgery, allowing their child to die rather than face inhumane institutional care at her fairly handicapped mental and functional level.

This case is tragic on a number of counts and is presented here as a possible morally legitimate exception, not the preferred norm. So-called "dying bins" or "warehouses" for the mentally retarded ought not exist, but de facto they do in many countries and some states, especially those whose finite budgets are tapped dry by many more vocal needs and lobbies. Societal funding is notoriously inadequate for institutional care or community-based programs for the severely deformed and mentally impaired. Frequently, they are the locus for budget cuts or freezes. Another tragic component is the fact that, for whatever reasons, the Novicks lack the personal resources—financial, psychic, and motivational—to accept responsibility for Betsy's care. In reality, the cost of lifetime care at home with professional assistance or in a reasonably humane facility may be astronomical, categorically beyond a given family's resources. The psychic "cost," especially of a bedridden, incontinent, perhaps non-responsive but non-terminal child, accumulates with the passage of years. In Betsy Novick's case, the medical, financial, psychic, and societal forces so coalesced to make nontreatment, with the prognosis of death (and eternal life to come), at least arguably one valid interpretation of her "quality of life"-based best interest.

Finally, one more case will be cited, one in which the infant patient, whom we will call Marie, had some minimal level of relational potential and was reasonably pain-free. In her case, social factors are presented as potentially tilting the scale from a presumed mandate for continued ventilator therapy to an optional, though not mandatory decision to "pull the plug." Marie was born to a teenage single mother, whose staunchly religious family disowned her for being pregnant and cast her out as "evil." The infant Marie was thought to have Sudden Infant

Death Syndrome. She was resuscitated and was then diagnosed as having some other neuromyopathy. Symptomatically she had sustained some asphyxia-induced brain damage, could not breathe unassisted, had central nervous system damage, and became flaccid (no body movement). Physicians noted, on the basis of observation across time, that Marie "could see," "she could perceive" and "she smiled," but "she never did very much more than that." Her middle and upper brain functions were severely impaired, but one pediatrician admitted that she was "kind of on the borderline" of any relational potential guideline. He suggested that Marie's level of interaction was comparable to that of higher animals, a beloved pet dog perhaps. Her caretakers generally fell into two groups, those who adopted her as a tragically afflicted, but "mascot-like" human person deserving life-prolongation via continued ventilated care and those who felt that such a barely relational, minimal human existence is not a quality or kind of life for the patient worth sustaining artificially. Both groups seemed to argue their positions as in Marie's best interest.

Medically, Marie would never breathe on her own and would never walk. Her brain damage was permanent and static. Financially, the cost of Marie's stay in the (N)ICU was roughly $1,000 per day and later hospital maintenance of her ventilator-dependent life would run approximately $700 per day. Marie's mother signed off as primary caretaker and decision-maker, refusing either to grant permission to cease ventilator care or to mandate continued aggressive therapy. As an ostracized, teenage, single parent she withdrew from the scene, unable to cope with the complexities and trauma of it all. At that point in time [mid-1970s] the hospital felt compelled to presume that Marie ought to be sustained on the ventilator and offered the best care possible to enhance her minimally conscious participation in the goods of life. Six and one-half years later, after an expenditure of at least $2,043,500, Marie was transferred from her hospital "home" to a new and less expensive chronic care facility.[15] Away from the sophisticated equipment of a pediatric ICU and acute care hospital, she "arrested" periodically and died, while still on a ventilator, six months later.

With all due respect for the commitment to life-prolongation of the institution and to the personal dedication of a number of individual staff persons, was it worth it for Marie's sake? Is respirator-dependent, barely "conscious," hospital-bound, quadriplegic existence, at a financial cost to "someone" of $700 to $1,000 per diem, a life worth living? Might it not be judged an excessive burden, if not to the patient in an isolated experiential sense, at least to the patient seen as part of her wider social milieu? Given the extremely minimal potential for her to physiologically experience life, to interact in any responsive way beyond an occasional grin, cannot the burdens of her immobile, ventilator-bound condition and the cost of such care, both financial and emotional, be brought to bear as indicators that "burden" may outweigh "benefit"?

As noted in the previous section of this chapter, one might approach such a case methodologically in either of two ways. One might establish some national, regional, or institutional policy that excludes, with rare exceptions, permanent ventilator-dependence or lifelong TPN on severely brain damaged patients as unacceptable qualities of life, prolonged by courses of treatment that exceed good medical practice. Such a macro-allocation or categorical decision would set up a generic limit which would forestall cases like Marie's lingering on unresolved. Perhaps a Hospital Review Committee or a court hearing should be procedurally programmed in to confirm whether a given patient is or becomes a member of this a priori excluded species of cases.

Or, as Paul Johnson would prefer, one might follow the pattern this author used above. Given the patient's borderline relational potential and static prognosis, given the generic and in some sense inordinate burden of permanent hospital residency and ventilator-dependence, and correlatively given the exorbitant daily drain on society's finite health care resources to sustain the child at such a barely conscious level, the infant-patient's total well-being—her physiological, psychological, social, and spiritual interests—may best be served by ceasing artificial respiration. In this schema social burden acts as a corroborating, possibly balance-tipping factor in determining patient well-being, but never as a lone criterion placed over against the total best interests of the non-competent handicapped newborn.

Final Comments

Before dotting the last "i" and crossing the final "t" in this lengthy volume, four concluding comments seem in order:

First, this author finishes this study humbled, both by the complexity of the ethical issues involved in nontreatment decision making and by the true scholarly acumen of all the ethicists surveyed and critiqued herein. My disagreements with Ramsey or Singer and Tooley or Reich or McCormick or Duff and Campbell in no way indicate a demeaning of their valid insights and contributions to the ongoing dialogue concerning when to accept or forego treatment. My own conclusions depend on and in many ways echo their collective wisdom.

Second, rarely are the controversial cases regarding the advisability of nontreatment as clear-cut or neatly defined as anencephaly **alone** or a Down's Syndrome baby whose **only** other anomaly is an easily correctable digestive blockage. More often than not a child with one so-called "handicap" is actually the victim of a complex of related conditions which affect multiple organ systems to varying degrees. For example, a newborn with spina bifida cystica must deal not only with a spinal hole and protruding sac of nerve tissue, but also with the CNS, renal, bowel, genital, and orthopedic complications related to the damaged tissue in the myelomeningocele. So also, the tendency toward obesity, the probability of hydrocephalus, and the possibility of mental retardation (usually minimal if shunted early) cannot be excluded from the amalgam of "spina bifida"-related burdens.

Then there is the real possibility in some instances that "the cure will be worse than the disease." Most notorious is the possibility that ventilator assistance for premature babies, which is essential to sustain respiration while allowing their underdeveloped lungs to mature, will itself cause chronic lung disease. The result may be permanent ventilator-dependence. In the same way, various drug therapies may in fact counteract one deficiency (e.g., low blood pressure and hemoglobin rates) at the price of causing another, perhaps more chronic medical problem (cardiomyopathy).

In other words, most handicapped infants suffer from multiple inter-related anomalies, which are not infrequently compounded by the very treatments intended to inhibit or arrest some symptoms. Dr. Anne Fletcher, Director of the NICU at Children's Hospital National Medical Center, suggests that such complex interdependent diagnoses/prognoses are most evident in the cases of severely asphyxiated babies, small "premies" with multiple immature organ systems, and infants who have contracted severe chronic lung disease while on a ventilator.[16] The neat, single function handicap, which would lend itself to clear ethical analysis, is rare. More often, diagnoses, prognoses, and projections of functional potential or deficits require multi-leveled, multi-factored judgment calls. "Handicapped newborns" is an umbrella term for infants usually afflicted with a series of congenital and therapy-related problems.

Lastly, eschewing a medical indications approach as too vitalistic, this author realizes that ethical decision making for nontreatment will inevitably incorporate transbiological factors related to the patient's well-being—suffering, inconvenience, relational potential, familial stress, societal resources, personal rights and responsibilities. With the introduction of values one is forced to confront philosophical and theological debates as to priorities and what is or is not in a given patient's holistic best interest. Prudence ought to be the operative virtue, coupled with a healthy mutual respect, both for the complexity of the calculus and the probable integrity of opponents who adopt a different hierarchy or prioritization of values. This is not to imply that all decisions are relative in a subjectivistic or libertarian sense. On the contrary, even in the "gray," there is the obvious distinction between "eggshell" and "charcoal." But as we move closer to those borderline cases, such as Babies Fred, Betsy, and Marie, it is well to acknowledge that neither alternative is wonderful, categorically life-enhancing. Both are fraught with burden and deficits. Opting for or against treatment in these cases becomes a tragic judgment, eliciting humility in the face of a diminished human life, whether treatment is accepted or foregone.

It has been the purpose of this volume to examine the various dimensions of being a person, of having life and living it to the fullest. Adopting a totality-based, multi-layered approach to a patient's well-being seems to be the safest guarantee that no neonatal patient's best interest for a full life will be overlooked or prematurely short-circuited. Projecting the quality of the newborn patient's life in terms of physiological, psychological, social, and spiritual potential, decision makers can then prudently choose to accept or forego treatment, always keeping the patient's well-being central. "To treat or not to treat?" should always remain a patient-centered, life-respecting question.

NOTES

[1]H. Richard Niebuhr, **Christ and Culture** (New York: Harper and Row, 1951); Avery Dulles, **Models of the Church** (Garden City: Doubleday and Company, 1974).

[2]Meilaender, "If This Baby Could Choose . . . " p. 317. See Chapter One for a fuller treatment of Meilaender's idea.

[3]Johnson, "Selective Nontreatment of Defective Newborns," pp. 39–53; Johnson, "Selective Nontreatment and Spina Bifida," pp. 91–111.

[4]For an entrance into the finite resource questions of costs, macro-allocation, and justice see "Medical Miracles—But How to Pay the Bill?" **Time** (10 December 1984), pp. 71–73, 77–80, 83–86; Stuart J. Kingma, "Mere Survival or a More Abundant Life?" **Ecumenical Review** 33 (July 1981), pp. 257–271; Robert Sade, "Is Health Care a Right?" **Image** 7 (1974), pp. 11–18; James F. Childress, "Priorities in the Allocation of Health Care Resources," **Soundings** 62 (Fall 1979), pp. 258–269; Victor R. Fuchs, **Who Shall Live? Health Economics and Social Choice** (New York: Basic Books, 1974); Fred Frohock, **Special Care: Medical Decisions at the Beginning of Life** (Chicago: University of Chicago Press, 1986), pp. 138ff.

[5]"The Hippocratic Oath," in **Encyclopedia of Bioethics**, p. 1731.

[6]Interview with Murray Pollack, M.D., Pediatric Intensivist, Children's Hospital National Medical Center, Washington, D.C., 18 April 1985.

[7]Robert M. Veatch, "The Technical Criteria Fallacy," **Hastings Center Report** 7 (August 1977), pp. 15–16.

[8]Interview with Anne Fletcher, M.D., Director of Neonatal Intensive Care Unit, Children's Hospital National Medical Center, Washington, D.C., 18 April 1985.

[9]For a list, description, and photographic analysis of these and other similarly death-dealing conditions a definitive source-book is David W. Smith, **Recognizable Patterns of Human Mal-**

formation, 3d ed. (Philadelphia: W.B. Saunders Company, 1982).

[10]Johnson, "Selective Nontreatment of Defective Newborns," p. 47.

[11]Voigtlander, **An Ethical Theory,** pp. 161–164.

[12]Richard E. Behrman, ed. **Neonatology, Diseases of the Fetus and Infant,** p. 591; as cited in Voigtlander, **An Ethical Theory,** p. 161.

[13]Ramsey, **Ethics at the Edges of Life,** p. 215.

[14]This case appears as Number 16 in Beauchamp and Childress, **Principles of Biomedical Ethics** (1979), pp. 265–266. Credit is given to Robert Veatch as the author of this case. For more information on Seckel syndrome see David W. Smith, **Recognizable Patterns of Human Malformation,** pp. 94–95.

[15]The dollar total was arrived at by two multiplications:

$1,000 (per day) × 1,277 days
    (3 and $1/2$ years in ICU) = $1,277,000
$ 700 (per day) × 1,095 days
    (3 years in hospital care) = $ 766,500
                                         $2,043,500

Other medical and care costs as well as the cost of Marie's time in the chronic care facility would still have to be added onto this figure.

[16]Interview with Anne Fletcher, M.D., 18 April 1985.

Author Index

Topic Index